Three Simple Steps to Flatten Your Belly

A trio of methods—**for men and women of virtually any age**—to help you reduce your stomach and to keep the fat off through exercise and a change in your eating habits.

By
CHET CUNNINGHAM

UNITED RESEARCH PUBLISHERS

First published in the United States of America in 1994

by United Research Publishers, P.O. Box 2344
Leucadia, California 92024,U.S.A.

Art Work by: Kevin Anderson, Cardiff-by-the-Sea, CA

Cover Design by: The Art Department, Encinitas, CA

Book Design & Typesetting by: The Final Draft,
Encinitas, CA

Library of Congress Catalog Card Number 94-060412

ISBN 0-961-49248-1

Printed in the United States of America

10 9 8 7 6 5 4 3 2 1

Dedicated to

Rose Marie Cunningham who is the driving force behind the pen, the inspiration behind the thoughts, the loving care and nurturing in all things, in all ways and at all times.

For all of this, I thank you.

NOTICE

This book is not intended to be a substitute or a replacement for medical advice or treatment of your eating habits or any weight problem that you may have. It is solely intended as an educational and informational book designed to acquaint the average layman with another look at weight problems, fat intake, and exercises that may help in flattening your stomach. Before starting this, or any other exercise or weight control program, be sure to check with your medical doctor to see if there is any element of this plan that could be harmful to you. If you have any back problems, be doubly certain to check with your doctor and get his approval of the exercises and the weight reduction program.

Order additional copies of this book from:

UNITED RESEARCH PUBLISHERS
P.O. Box 2344
Leucadia, CA 92024 U.S.A.

Full 30-day money-back guarantee if not satisfied

CONTENTS

The four abdominal muscle groups
How your body works
How about those magic spot reducing machines?
A look at exercise machines
Devices, ideas that don't work
Can you sweat off fat?

The three step program
Varicose veins
Back pain
Hernia
Constipation

The look of muscles
No pain — no gain — no way!
Some exercises we won't be doing
Your commitment
Ready, exercise...No, hold it, warm-up first

The basic first eight exercises

STEP TWO
Burning Off The Fat

STEP THREE
Low-fat Eating

INTRODUCTION

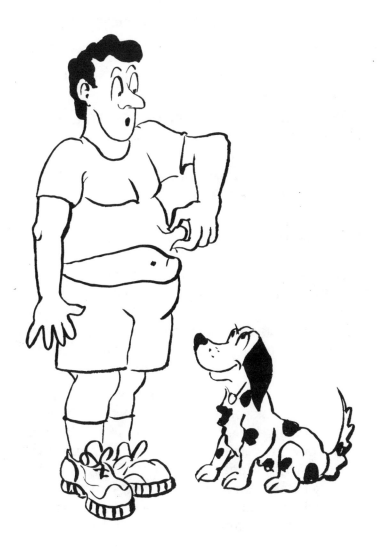

"What a gut!"

"My dear, she simply never should wear a knit dress. Look at the size of that tummy pouching out."

"Look at that guy's mid forties paunch!"

"I've seen beer bellies before but, nothing like that!"

"I'm not going to the beach again until I can flatten my tummy. It was embarrassing."

Ever heard comments like these before? Ever had the same thing said about you? Ever wished that you could get rid of your own "gut" and flatten out that belly to the hard, washboard look that your stomach used to have when you were 21?

YOU CAN DO IT

Yes, that's what I said. You <u>can flatten your stomach.</u> There's no magic to it. There is no wonder pill you can take, no chance that a spot reducing exercise or machine can shimmy, rock or roll off the pounds under your belt line. There is in short no simple way to change the contours of your body.

Let's say you're 33 and you have a roll around the old middle. It took you ten years to put it there. It won't come off in ten easy lessons. If you're 45 or 55 or 66, man or woman, the same principal holds true. It took you years to "earn" that kind of a belly—and it's going to take you some hard work, some discipline and an important change in your eating habits to get that fat off your stomach and sides and to keep it off.

I'm glad you're interested in giving it a try, otherwise you wouldn't have read this far. Let's get it right out in the open so there will be no surprises, no recriminations, no easy excuses if you backslide and dump the program.

Let's answer some questions right here. No, this program will not turn you into a muscle bound weight lifter ready to challenge Hulk Monster Man in the WWF. What we're talking about here is a way to flatten your stomach, and at the same time cut excess weight off many other parts of your body as well.

Yes, the male body does store excess fat in the stomach and side area, those old love handles. It's natural and happens to every man. That doesn't mean the blubber has to stay there.

Women put on a lot of weight around their hips and thighs as well as the stomach. This program will help burn off those fat cells all over your body. You win all kind of ways.

"Hey, what about those spot reducing machines and lotions and gimmicks you see advertised? Won't one of them work to get rid of my belly?" Sorry, Geraldine, those spot reducing gadgets reduce only one thing, your bank account. They simply don't work to eliminate one body area of fat cells. If there's enough aerobic exercise associated with their use, they can help reduce overall body fat a little, but experts on physical culture say those spot reducing gadgets are a waste of money.

"I'm 55, what can this program do for me?" The answer here is: it can do wonders. If you're 55, or 45 or 65, the program works the same. It will produce results in direct proportion to your involvement in it. If you work all three steps at the same time, the excess fat cells will get burned up just as they will on a 20 year old stock clerk or a 35 year old sitting down all day secretary. You work at it, do your aerobics and eat good healthy low-fat meals, and you'll see results quickly.

Any more questions? Good, so let's move on.

TEST YOUR BELLY BULGE QUOTIENT

Do you really need to work on your stomach? Let's do a self-evaluation here. Try the old pinch test. You've probably done this before. Relax, let your belly fall into its usual place, then grab that area just below your belly button and pinch.

Can you get a roll of fat between your thumb and finger of more than an inch? If so, you need this program. This applies to men or women. Move around to your sides and try the pinch test again. More men will have a roll here than women. Try the pinch test all over your abdomen, midriff, sides, back.

If there's more than an inch between thumb and finger, you are a prime candidate for this three step program.

Doctors will use calipers and do the same thing for a fat fee. A little play on words there. The caliper test is recognized by most authorities as a good way to judge the amount of body fat that a person is carrying.

If you find more than an inch of fat down there or on the sides, it simply means that you're eating more fatty foods than your body is burning off. The excess, the net, is saved by our efficient bodies and stored in various places, the tummy for most men and the hips and thighs and arms for many women.

Later on in this book we'll tell you how to counter this problem and start burning off those extra fat cells.

THE TAPE MEASURE TEST

Another way to test yourself for a bulging tummy is simpler. All you have to do is undress and stand sideways in front of a full length mirror. See anything you don't like? Is that bulge in your tummy too much even to pull in anymore?

How much have you changed in the past ten years? What did you look like when you were 20 or 30, or 40? If your present appearance is lumpy, poochy, bulging and paunchy, you are a good student for the old university of flattening the tummy.

Find a cloth tape measure. If you're male, your wife might have one in a sewing kit or in her make up cabinet. Now take off your shirt and measure your chest. Be sure you take a big breath to expand your chest to its fullest. Then measure around it just under your armpits. The tape should be pulled snug and be flat and not twisted. Mark that measurement down on your notepad. Say it's 38.

Now, let your stomach relax. Don't push it out or suck it in, just normal. Measure your waist at your navel.

Again, keep the tape snug, not too tight and be sure it's flat and not twisted.

If your waist measurement is 33 and your chest 38, you're in better shape than you thought. For a man, the chest measurement should be five inches greater than his waist. On women the difference should be ten inches. For example a chest measurement of 38 would require a waist measurement of 28.

If a man's chest measures 42 and his waist 42, guess who needs this program?

If a woman's chest measurement is 36 and her waist is 34, she, too is in need of some belly reduction.

TRY THE POKE TEST

If you want more proof that you need this three step program, try the poke test. On this one we're going to take one finger and poke it into your tightened stomach, abdomen or waist.

Did you lose your finger in there somewhere? If it sinks out of sight before it hits your muscle girdle, you need some exercise help.

Many a stomach sags and bulges simply because of weak abdominal muscles. These muscles are some of the least used in our body. Most of us don't use them when we walk, work or play. They get lazy, fat and flabby and if there's a pot belly of accumulated fat, they give way easily to accommodate the extra weight and size and your protruding belly gets larger and poochier by the year.

Part of the purpose of the abdominal muscles is to hold some of your internal organs in place. The weaker these muscles become, the more apt it is that some of those organs will move enough to cause you some stress. They often slip and slide just enough to make a change in a person's posture. This will further aggravate the problem of the stomach muscles and they will weaken again and more fat arrives to help and the internal organs have a little more room to wander around. Not a good happening.

The only way to counteract these problems is by exercising and strengthening those abdominal muscles. We'll explain later just what muscles these are, where they lay in your abdomen and what their jobs are.

YES, VIRGINIA, THERE ARE DIFFERENT BODY TYPES

"Oh, I'm not fat it's just my body type. My mother is the same way."

"He eats like a horse and never gains a pound. I hate him. How can he do that?"

Both the statements above are true to a degree. The first one is a favorite ploy of the perpetually overweight person, one we're not concerned with in this book. However, both do have some bearing on the current topic.

There are different body types. Many experts today have settled on three basic body types, regardless if you're male or female.

These are the mesomorph, the ectomorph and the endomorph.

The mesomorph is the athletic type, big boned and muscular, the football captain, president of the class type. His body is more hard and rugged than most. This man or woman is often of moderate height with a long neck and broad shoulders and a large chest. His waist may be narrower with broad hips.

This man or woman can excel in sports where agility, endurance, strength and power are essential, but probably will put on considerable weight once their playing days are over.

This weight responds well to exercise and aerobic workouts and muscle tone often returns quickly.

The endomorph, on the other hand, often is smaller than normal, has little muscle development and tends to be soft and round with a lot of weight centered around his mid section.

This endomorph type often is poor to terrible in athletics that take agility, power and strength. If he or she is athletic it is in a skill type activity such as golf, archery or swimming.

When an endomorph tries to lose weight or slim down a pot belly, he or she often is faced with a slow track operation. The stomach may never slim down to an ideal washboard, simply due to the general shape and form of the individual.

The ectomorph type body is usually on the fragile side being thin-boned and often tall. The person's neck, legs and arms are all long but the trunk usually on the short side.

Little fat ever clings to this type person. He or she is the "poor feeder" as the cattlemen say. They can eat anything and never gain weight. Many ectomorphs have poor posture because of their light muscular system to hold them in correct alignment.

A program such as this to strengthen the abdominal muscles on this type body will usually produce excellent results and rather quickly. There's less to burn off and the muscular strengthening through exercising can produce the washboard stomach.

Now, with this much background, let's move on to the plan to cut down on your overactive belly.

This is the *Three Simple Steps to Flatten Your Belly* book and here are the three procedures you can use to help reclaim a harder, flatter belly.

Step 1: Learn how your abdomen is constructed, which muscles hold you together, and then start an exercise program that will help strengthen and tighten those muscles. A fifteen minute workout here can do wonders, even three times a week. Five times a week will bring quicker results. Anything you do on this phase of the program is better than nothing at all.

Step 2: The abdominal exercises will do little to reduce your belly. They are designed to strengthen and tighten those muscles. Reducing that stomach is the purpose of step two: to initiate an aerobic exercise workout. This program might be walking, jogging, swimming, skating, canoeing, bicycling, aerobic dancing or one of many other forms of exercise except lifting weights that is kept up continuously.

The longer you walk or run the better. You might start out at fifteen minutes and build up gradually to thirty minutes without a rest. The experts say a thirty minute walk, jog, swim or bicycling without rest is the ideal time. Here again any aerobic workout you can do three, or five times a week will help you just that much more. This is the exercise that will burn the fat cells off your body, all over your body and will begin the task of reducing the roll around your middle.

Step 3: A new approach to eating. Both of the above steps will do little to reduce your belly unless you begin a new regimen of limiting the amount of fat you eat daily. The low-fat method of eating is a natural and healthful way to get your daily supply of energy, and at the same time not over load your diet with fat.

When your body burns up more fat than you input, it means you have a negative balance, and your body starts to burn down those fat cells where it had stored more fat than you had been burning in your sedentary life. It can be an exciting and interesting change in eating habits for you that will help you stay healthier for the rest of your life.

There it is, the three step program. I told you it wasn't going to be easy -- but neither is it impossibly hard. What it takes is your own determination and will power to start and stay with the program until you begin to see results. Then that will fire your enthusiasm to continue the three steps until you've reached your goal.

Once you get to your goal, you'll switch to a maintenance program that cuts down the exercises and the aerobics and maintains the low-fat diet to keep you trim and beautiful.

DOES IT ALL WORK?

You bet! This program is balanced, reasonable, logical, physically applicable and designed for the average man or woman who wants to trim his or her belly.

No magic elixirs, no wondrous reducing creams, no fantastic spot reducing machines. This is a simple and workable approach to cutting down on your body fat, and tightening your stomach muscles to get that flat belly look.

It is only designed to do stomach tightening and reduction.

It is not formulated to build bulging biceps, or massive shoulders, or thunder thighs.

Actually if you do a lot of weight room work to build up your stomach muscles, you could at the same time be increasing, not decreasing the size of your belly. How? Stomach muscles are thin and long, not massive as in your thighs or arms. They will increase in size little, but when they do, that exercise will not reduce the fat on your stomach muscles. The end result could be a belly even larger than before you did the stomach muscle building workouts.

This program doesn't attempt to build your stomach muscles, only to tighten and strengthen them, but at the same time it does reduce the amount of fat in your system, and around your midsection.

Game to give it a try?

You've bought the book already, so you might as well invest some of your time, sweat and good judgement and get on with the Three Step Program. Turn the page and move ahead to Step One:

STEP ONE

YOUR EXERCISE PROGRAM

Three Steps to Flatten Your Belly

Chapter 1
MUSCLES AND MACHINES AND HEALTH

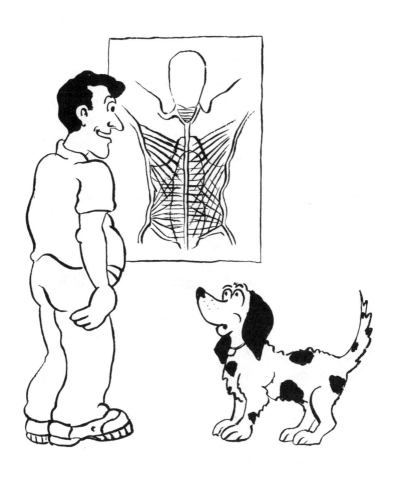

Let's get right to the guts of the problem. You have a slightly overactive belly and you want to do something about it. First we need to set up the ground rules, get some definitions out of the way and in general get you on board so you know enough about how your torso is put together so you understand how it works.

Some physical therapists consider the muscles that surround the torso in front as a form of a girdle. It isn't a bad description. These muscles form a network that holds you in place, that keeps your internal organs in their proper location and helps you to turn and twist and move any direction that you want to without any pain. Quite a mechanical device.

One minor drawback. If these muscles don't get exercised enough, they tend to lose their strength and ability to do their job. They get soft and stretch and generally let your body down and your belly push out and can cause all sorts of back aches and strains and pains.

The exercise these abdominal muscles need is not like that for any other muscle group in your body. You're not building up bulk muscle as you would working out your shoulders or your biceps for example. What your stomach muscles don't need is weight training. No grunting and groaning with the iron for the tummy. They need special exercises that we'll demonstrate on down the line.

You don't want your belly muscles to go bad on you. That's part of what we're going to touch on here. Some more details about this girdle that surrounds you.

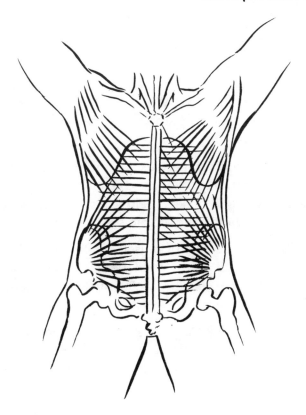

THE FOUR ABDOMINAL MUSCLE GROUPS

There are four groups of muscles that form this girdle around the front of your torso.

The rectus abdominis muscle is really one long muscle that covers your upper and lower abdomen and runs vertically from your rib cage down to your pubic bone. These are the sets of muscles that when properly conditioned can give a man's stomach that washboard effect. These are some of the muscles that help you do sit ups and are tremendously important.

The external oblique muscles run diagonally across the body from the lower ribs to the rectus abdominis muscles. These are what allow the body to rotate the trunk and flex the torso. When these muscles are in firm, hard condition they make the sides of your body look sleek and trim.

The internal oblique muscles are under the external obliques and run diagonally and at nearly right angles to the external. It makes a closely placed mesh of muscles that hold your body in firm control.

Both the oblique sets of muscles help the body to twist and turn and also control the size of your waistline. The sharper these muscles angle across each other, the narrower your waistline.

The traverse abdominis muscles run horizontally across your stomach. These are the workers that help to pull in your lower stomach and are some of the ones that will be worked on in the exercise portion of your program.

Now, surprise, but fat does have a place in your body makeup. All around these abdominal muscles, and those in the rest of your body, fat cells gather to act as insulation and cushioning for the muscles and the organs behind them. Fat is needed. The problem comes when too much fat accumulates and the muscles sag and nobody gets the work of the day done.

Two other muscles, not really in the stomach area, are important in these coming exercises. They are the psoas major and the iliacus muscles. The psoas goes from your thigh bone to the spinal column. The iliacus joins the hip and thigh bones. The two acting together help you to flex your thighs and to rotate the thigh outward.

HOW YOUR BODY WORKS

Think of your body as a production machine. Let's say you need 20 bitcus of energy to run your machine for normal, routine activity. You take in 20 bitcus and your burn off 20 bitcus of energy during the 24-hour period. Your mass remains the same.

However, you get lazy and start taking on more energy, you jump your intake to 30 bitcus of energy material a day, but still you only burn off 20 bitcus of that fuel. What happens? Your efficient body says, great, I'll just save that extra amount of bitcus for later use. So the body transforms that extra energy into fat cells and lodges them around your body.

This is exactly what happens when you eat more than your body needs, and when you eat more fat calories than your body can burn off. It settles to your waist, your tummy, your hips or thighs. The hips and thighs part is especially true for you women.

How do you get rid of the extra fat cells and the bulge they create on your belly, your arms, your hips and thighs? You do two things. One, you begin limiting your fat intake to slightly less than your body needs. Your efficient body machine remembers where those extra fat cells are, and they are called into service and used up to complete the 20 units needed. Your body is starting to lose those fat cells and weight, and your stomach and other fatty parts of your body will start to shrink.

The other way you work on those extra units of fat energy cells you intake, is to do more work. You set up an aerobics program of 20-30 minutes a day to burn off an extra ten units a day, when you are putting only 20 units into your system.

Your smart body knows where to go get those extra fat cells it needs to burn for energy and you are on your way to eliminating that bulging stomach and other fatty buildup areas. But don't look for results over night. It took you ten years to put on that bulge. Give it a three month workout and then take another look at the old belly.

The stomach exercises? How do they fit in? When this fat load begins to shrink, you need to exercise and strengthen those stomach muscles to jerk them back into their once tight and svelte appearance. If you reduce your belly without the exercises, the loose muscles will still be there and you won't notice as much difference. You need all three steps of this program for a complete practical belly reducing regimen.

HOW ABOUT THOSE MAGIC SPOT REDUCING MACHINES?

Lots of luck.

Our world today is hooked on "fast." We have fast food, fast access to news, fast communications, fast fax machines, fast computers, fast growing up, fast love.

Even with all this "fast" around, there is no fast way to lose weight or reduce you stomach bulge. It took you years to grow that pot belly, and it's going to take lots of hard work and effort on your part to get it off.

We're back to the three step program: exercise, fat burn-off and a change in eating habits. That's how to reduce your belly.

No machine or device can do all of these. Very few of them will help you burn off fat, none of them will help you restructure your eating program.

The only way to lose weight and flatten your stomach is by burning off more fat calories than you ingest.

Five machines might help you here, if you utilize them into the aerobic time frames where they will do you some good. They are treadmills, stair climbers, skiing machines, rowing machines and stationary bicycles. None of the machines that roll or massage you can possibly reduce or flatten your stomach.

If some machine or gadget claims that it will do all the work for you, and help you reduce weight and inches, jump away as fast as you can. Your body, your muscles must do the work to do you any good, not the machine.

A LOOK AT EXERCISE MACHINES

Today exercise equipment, gyms, personal trainers, machines, home gym equipment and hundreds of "devices" to help people reduce weight and stay in shape is a multi billion dollar market. With such a huge market comes the old line firms that produce fine equipment. Right along with them sweep in a host of quick buck artists who charge into this ready market with big claims, hot advertising programs, big busted girls in workout costumes and merchandise that is questionable at best and down right misleading at the worst.

Let's take a look at some of the equipment in relation to flattening your stomach:

The ones that can do you the most good to flatten your stomach are the machines that are designed for 20 to 30 minutes use at a session which will help you burn off fat.

These machines include the stationary cross country ski machines. These produce an aerobic effect if you use them long enough, and at the same time can be beneficial to other muscle groups as well.

The stair climber is totally exhausting, but if you utilize it at a level where you can maintain its use over a 20 minute period, it will produce the needed aerobic benefits of fat burning. This machine will also give you other muscle benefits.

The treadmill is another device that is excellent as an aerobic exercise. Most can be set at various speeds for walking, jogging or running, and will produce the related benefits. Walking has been described as the perfect aerobic exercise since it is not so exhausting that it can't be maintained for a half hour to several hours, and it does not produce the pressure and shocks that running does.

The secret here as with all of these aerobic machines, is that they give top benefit when used daily, and if that is not possible, then they should be used at aerobic level timed workout of 20 to 30 minutes four times a week.

The most common exercise machine today is probably the stationary bicycle. This device looks like a bicycle without a rear wheel. It has a chain and pedals and seat. The chain goes to the front wheel which is a flywheel of sorts that has a system to allow braking pressure to be applied to the front wheel to increase or decrease the amount of effort needed to pedal. Many such devices have computerized workout programs, can simulate hills and flats and various levels of stress. Some are high cost equipment, but the simple ones with just a mechanical brake and 15-minute timer are relatively inexpensive.

The exercise bike provides the simplest, least expensive and best form of fat burning exercise that most people can use.

The last of these aerobic exercise machines we're going to look at is a rowing machines. Not as popular today as they once were, the rower can be set at a stress level that will let you work it for the needed 20 minutes to hit your fat burning requirement.

Some drawbacks here. This machine is not recommended for people with high blood pressure, heart disease or some types of back problems.

Making a comeback in the device end of exercise equipment are the rubber cord stretchers. These are simply elastic pieces of rubber ropes with loops at each end. There are dozens of ways to use these stretchers being held by the hands and feet. These devices are mainly used for muscle workouts and don't help you lose any weight around your stomach. Use those in your next program to strengthen certain muscles.

A jump rope is a simple, inexpensive and worthwhile piece of equipment to help you flatten your stomach. They come in all sizes and types. For best results use your jump rope for 20 to 30 minutes a session at least four times a week. Some jump ropes come with instruction booklets. Here is one place there is no reason to buy a device. You can make a practical jump rope from clothes line rope or any piece of quarter inch rope.

DEVICES, IDEAS THAT DON'T WORK

While it's essential that you know what will work to help you flatten your stomach, it's also good to know what simply can't do you any good in this area. Here are some of them.

There are dozens of vibrating and massaging machines on the market today that have absolutely no value when it comes to flattening your stomach. Rollers, massaging equipment, vibrating chairs, belts and pads all might relax you and give you a fine feeling, but they won't reduce your body fat.

Hydromassage units, not as popular today as in the past. These units direct streams of water with some force on the body where the fat reduction is desired. The only benefit here is psychological, you'll relax and maybe soak out some aches and pains, but you definitely won't get any weight loss from a hydromassage.

Not used much anymore are the belt vibrators. These straps and machine powered shakers were supposed to vibrate fat off your muscles and it then would be passed out of your body. Wishful thinking that fooled a lot of people a long time.

You've heard of cellulite, that fatty material just under the skin and gives a dimpled effect to the skin. Medical specialists say there is nothing unusual about this storage of fat. It simply has a different effect on some people. The problem usually occurs in women.

There is no special program to get rid of cellulite. Most experts in the field say to work on a good weight reduction program and better eating habits and aerobic exercising and the cellulite fat will shrink and go away as well as any other fatty area of your body.

CAN YOU SWEAT OFF FAT?

Sweat suits may have originated not to keep an athlete warm during practice, but actually to help him or her sweat more to lose weight. Now experts agree that there is no such thing as losing fat from your body by sweating.

All sweating does is work water out of your system through the sweat glands. If you sweat off five pounds during a tough basketball game, you'll put that five pounds on the next day or two as you drink your normal amount of water.

Steam rooms were thought for years to be the place for rich old men and women to steam away pounds and pounds. Here the same sweat situation comes into play. You sweat out water in a steam room, not fat, and the next day the water is returned to the body and you weigh as much as you ever did.

The same holds true for the sauna. In the hot dry atmosphere you'll sweat and sweat and sweat. But you're only losing water from your system, water you need to survive, and no fat is boiling out through your pores.

Chapter 2
HEALTHY STOMACH MUSCLES

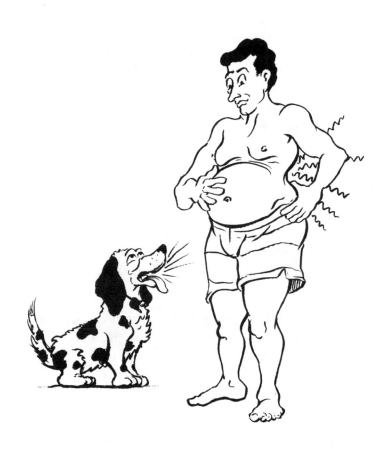

THE THREE STEP PROGRAM

Which brings us right back to the main theme of this book. The only way you can reduce your weight is by burning off the fat inside your body through aerobic exercises, and by cutting down on your overall intake of food, with a special emphasis on eating low-fat foods.

So far, so good. You've heard about the three steps to flatten your belly and what you need to do to change your physique. You've seen how a healthy stomach can do a lot to help hold your body in good posture and help in body movements. We've talked about those wild claims about machines and gimmicks that can't possibly help you flatten your stomach.

Now, let's move on to more reasons that you need a healthily muscled stomach. How? Just read on.

Whether you're 64 or 24 you still need a well maintained stomach simply because it can help your health in so many ways. So you don't want to show off a washboard belly at muscle beach come summertime. That flattened stomach is going to reward you in a number of other ways.

When men had to charge through the boulders and forests and slew the beasts for food, man had a good workout every day. The women in the cave also had to scrounge for roots and nuts and berries and wash their animal skin clothing in the nearby stream and chase after the kids and fight off the wild dogs.

In our modern world we have it too easy. Machines and electronic chips do most of the work for us these days. That's why it's so important to fight the good fight in the tummy bulge campaign.

Let's take a look at several of the health problems that a big belly can cause even if you don't know about them. They can sneak up on you before you understand what's happening.

VARICOSE VEINS

Did you realize that varicose veins can be caused and aggravated by weak stomach muscles? It's true. That's not the only condition that can cause varicose veins, but it's one of them.

Weak and flabby stomach muscles can get to the point where they aren't strong enough to hold some of your vital organs, such as your stomach, intestines, pancreas, liver and so on, in the right position inside your body. Often this means these organs can press against the abdominal wall and gravitate downward.

When this happens the out of normal position weight puts pressure on the large veins that return blood from your legs. It's like a tourniquet around those veins and it can impede and slow down the flow of blood back to your heart. This makes the blood slow down and it can collect in areas it shouldn't. That can enlarge the veins and push them toward the skin so they show through and even bulge.

By taking care of your belly, you can prevent one cause of varicose veins. Whether you're 54 or 34, varicose veins is one condition that you don't want to have.

BACK PAIN

Many general practitioner doctors these days see a lot of patients with back pain. This is often more frequent with older patients, but can strike anyone.

A great deal of the pain in the lower back is related to muscle use and disuse. Some of the most important sets of muscles that affect the back are the stomach area ones.

Weak stomach muscles can add to any other back problem, can probably be the cause of certain back pains, and the lack of use of stomach muscles through inactivity, can be another cause of your back pain.

Dr. Fred Geisler, is a neurosurgeon who heads the Comprehensive Spine Care Center at Columbus Hospital's Chicago Institute for Neurosurgery and Neuroresearch. He says that when people put on added weight in the stomach area, it causes problems with the back.

"Then the musculature is not balanced. If you put on extra weight in your abdomen, this is carrying you forward. Your abdominal muscles, which hold the anterior portion of your spine straight, are not that functional and competent. That puts you into poor posture, puts stress on the bones themselves and causes them to deteriorate."

So, the idea here is that by strengthening your stomach muscles all over the "girdle" of intermeshed muscles, you can help your stomach and at the same time do good things for your back. As you gradually lose weight from your stomach, your body will have a better chance to function normally, you should develop better posture and reduce the problems of lower back pain.

One of the reasons for a strong stomach is that a weak one will help to throw your body posture the wrong position. If you have added weight in the stomach area, it can make your pelvis drop in front and raise in back. This can cause a swayback problem that can put added strain on your back and squeeze the vertebrae which can in turn pressure the nerves that run through that area and cause you one nasty lower back pain.

So the good old strong stomach muscles can help you again here by keeping your posture in better shape, eliminating those misalignments of the pelvis and spine and reduce or avoid that low back pain.

HERNIA

It doesn't happen often, but a weakened stomach muscle girdle can lead to hernia problems. A hernia is when a part of your stomach or intestine pushes out through the muscles of your abdominal wall. The pain is memorable and usually surgery is required to repair the puncture.

Hernias can occur after a intense fit of sneezing or coughing, or a great strain when you are lifting something you probably shouldn't be lifting in the first place.

If your stomach muscles are strong, they hold all of those organs firmly in place. But when the strain comes, and there is a weak spot in your mesh of stomach muscles, the organ can burst out through it and cause all sorts of problems.

A firm, hard stomach will help hold all of those organs tightly in place and avoid any chance of a hernia.

CONSTIPATION

Weak stomach muscles can contribute to poor elimination and the chance of constipation. Those weak muscles will let your organs move out of their normal position. This added pressure and weight can lead to abnormal twists and turns in your intestines. In some cases enough weight can almost pinch close the intestine the way you do when you bend a water hose to shut off the water.

Weak stomach muscles can also have less of a beneficial effect of helping food to move along your lower digestive tract.

Those exercises to help you get a strong stomach wall will do you a lot more good than just create that hard flat belly.

Now, we have the preliminaries covered, let's get on with the meat of the program in step one, your personal workout to start flattening your stomach. Just proceed to chapter three.

Chapter 3
STARTING YOUR EXERCISE PROGRAM

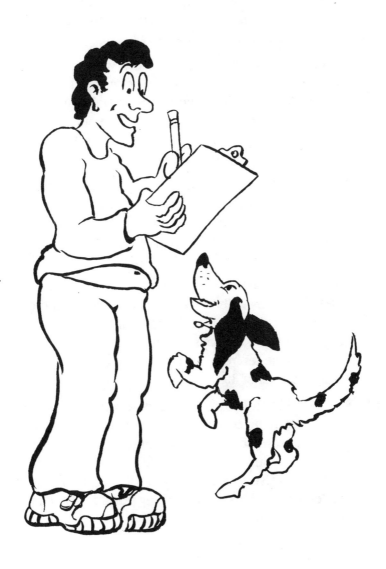

All right, so far. We're getting there. This is the chapter where we start your exercise program. Before we plunge right in, we need to define a few terms and set up some ground rules.

To communicate effectively, we all need to be on the same page, understand the terminology that is being used. Let's get that out of the way first.

ROUTINE: This term refers to all of the workouts and exercises that are done for a given body part. There is a routine for you to do if you want to build up your shoulders and pecs and another one for your biceps. In this book we're talking about a routine for your abdominal muscles and that's all.

EXERCISE: Here we mean any proscribed movement that is done to improve or strengthen any individual body part. This abdominal routine contains a variety of exercises such as leg raises, shoulder crunches, cross-overs and side curl ups.

SET: This means that the exercise will be done a specific number of times without resting. For example if the instructions call for ten repetitions of the leg raises that will be a set. If it says do three sets, that means you will do the ten repetitions of the leg raises three times, or a total of 30.

REPS, REPETITIONS: This is the completion of one exercise from the beginning and back to the starting point. For example on a double knee raise you lie on the floor on your back, bring your knees up to your chest, then raise them so your body forms an "L," then lower your legs to the starting position. That's a rep on the double knee raise.

REST: This is the time between sets that you get a small break, from half a minute to a minute to let your body recoup a little. Don't get distracted and rest too long as this will lessen the effectiveness of the exercise.

THE LOOK OF MUSCLES

Let's talk a minute about muscles and how they appear.

MUSCLE MASS: This simply means how large a muscle is. The stomach muscles are small in comparison to other body muscles. The biceps or the calf muscles for example. That's why we don't use weights in these exercises. But the stomach muscles do need more reps for optimum strength and development.

MUSCULARITY: This word means the contrast between muscle and fatty tissue. Right now your stomach muscles probably have more fatty tissue between around and in front of them than there is muscle. That's what we want to change and bring up the muscularity ratio so we can feel and see the difference and have a flatter, harder belly.

DEFINITION: A term more used in muscle building than in body health talk. This means how good the muscle looks under the skin. This is easy to see on biceps not so easy to see on your stomach. The longer you use this routine and the more fatty tissue is burned off your belly, the better you will be able to see the definition of those stomach muscles that we're strengthening with the routines and the better low-fat eating habits.

MUSCLE ACTION

FLEX: This term simply means to contract a muscle. When you pick up a glass or a fork, certain muscles flex so you can perform this task. When you flex muscles in an exercise to move a leg or shoulder, your muscles in that area flex to do the work. When you double the effort and consciously squeeze that muscle as hard as possible, it is said that you are putting the muscle in a peak contraction. This helps the muscle even more than simply flexing it.

PEAK CONTRACTION: This is that time when you squeeze a muscle as hard as you can, it goes far beyond simply flexing the muscle. On all of your exercises you should try for peak contraction, squeezing those used muscles as much as possible to extend and multiply the value of the exercise.

STRETCH: The stretch position of a muscle is when it is the opposite of flexed. Then it is relaxed. Bring one fist up to your shoulder and flex your muscle. When you let your hand return to your side and open your fingers, those muscles are in the stretched position.

ANY PAIN - NO GAIN - NO WAY!

No pain, no gain? Forget it. We're not tearing up muscles in clean and jerk here. This is a stomach flattening routine and pain is the last thing we want.

You're doing this routine so you can look and feel better and be healthier. It makes no sense to have to endure pain and aches and problems—with the hope that you might feel better later. Forget that no pain no gain stuff. Now, you just might be a little bit stiff after a workout, especially the first few times, but that's not pain. That's just a little minor inconvenience so you can get past the beginner's syndrome and into the real workouts.

There are four main hallmarks of a good exercise program:

1. Workout on a comfortable mat, padded bench or low table made for exercising. A lot of abdominal exercises are done lying down or sitting up. Any serious exercising done on a hard floor will soon leave you so sore and bruised you won't want to get started the second day. For the lying down exercises, a mat or two or three heavy blankets folded will do the job. For the sitting down ones, a pillow or folded towel or blanket will help.

2. Throw out any exercises that can hurt you. If you have a sore or bad back, don't do any exercises that will aggravate it. I bought a rowing machine once and felt proud that I did a hundred rowing motions on it. The next morning when I tried to get out of bed I couldn't straighten my back. I waddled around all day before I could straighten up. I never used that rowing machine again.

The same can be true on certain exercises that "good backs" can tolerate. No exercises to help the abdomen that can hurt your back or aggravate any back problem will be used in this book.

3. Don't go over your limit. Know how much you can exercise and don't go ballistic and do a hundred reps when you should be doing two sets of ten. Even if you want to see dramatic results, the slow approach will be a longer lasting one. Hot and heavy at the start will soon burn out or end in pain and frustration, avoidance of the program and your having the same bulging belly come swim suit time this spring.

4. Take a break between sets and exercises. If you're puffing after the first set on any exercise, be sure to take a small break before you start the next set. That's why they're broken up into sets instead of saying do 50 reps. After one exercise don't charge right into the next. Stand up, move around, run in place, do some breathing exercises, skip a little rope. Then go back to the next exercise. Don't rush. Don't try to do a whole series of belly exercises in a row, such as bent knee sit ups, V seats and a rowing exercise. If you do you stand a good chance to overwork those muscles in too short a time and you'll be sore and angry the next day.

By overworking one day, you won't be able to do the needed number of reps or sets the next day. Take it easy, stay within your ability and your development, and stay exercising for the long pull.

SOME EXERCISES WE WON'T BE DOING

Yes, there are three excellent exercises that will help firm and support and strengthen your abdomen, but we won't be doing those in this routine. You see, we want you to trim and flatten your belly, but we don't want you to blow out your back and put you in traction or worse.

That's why we're ignoring three of the best exercises and concentrating on the others, so you don't hurt your back. Nearly half of the adult population complain about back pains, back ache or go to their doctor for back pain problems.

Too many. So, that includes half of you reading this book. We don't want to make your back any worse, and these three exercises wouldn't have any way of making your back stronger. Another series of back exercises might do that, but right now we're worried about your belly.

So we won't be doing three exercises. We'll spell them out so you'll know. If you're 21, hard as a satellite re-entry cone, and gung ho, go ahead and do them. For the rest of us, don't bother, we'll get to the same point, even if a little slower, but with greater safety.

Oh, if you have any qualms at all about doing a specific exercise or even starting this program, be sure to check with your doctor first. Show it to him and see if he thinks you're fit enough to do the routine.

Now, for those three exercises.

Straight-leg sit-ups   Most experts say this is the toughest exercise you can do to give the greatest benefit to your stomach muscles. Sit-ups done this way, with your legs flat and straight on the floor means that the iliopsoas muscles from your spinal column to your thigh bone do most of the work.

This isn't what you need for your stomach. Also when the hip flexors are used in this exercise, the pelvis tilts forward and the muscles in the lower back are contracted and can give you a swayback condition. The more you do sit-ups the more they can shorten the muscles in the lower back and thighs and cause more forward pelvis tilt.

In short it can give your back a giant pain if you already have some backaches and pains. So forget about straight leg sit-ups.

The solution is to bend your knees when you do sit-ups. Do this and put your toes under some heavy furniture and this throws the work of doing these modified sit-ups into your stomach muscles where we want it. This almost eliminates any problems for your back. But if you try the bent leg sit up and your back still hurts, simply quit that exercise and substitute another one for it.

Short leg lifts   This is another classic exercise with the victim lying flat on his back and lifting the legs six inches off the floor and holding them there.

This one can really kill your back, even if it's strong and firm to begin with. The problem is most of us aren't strong enough to hold our legs off the floor that way for long. When our stomach muscles give out we compensate by lifting the lower back off the floor. That means a forward rotation of the pelvis which aggravates your lower back and leads to more trouble.

Therefore, forget about this exercise. It's simply too hard on anyone, and if you have a sensitive back, don't even think about the short leg lift.

Standing toe touch   This is the third exercise we won't be doing. For this you stand with feet two feet apart and arms extended to your sides. Then you bend and touch right hand to left toe. The result is a lot of gravity working as your bend forward and it does little for your stomach muscles.

This is one of the exercises some suggest for strengthening the muscles in the lower back, but if you strain and bounce to get to that toe, you can cause more harm than good.

So forget about the standing toe touch.

YOUR COMMITMENT

To do the most good, you should commit yourself to a regular program of exercise from three to five times a week. Five times is better, but with three times you'll see progress. The harder you work at the exercises the more good they will do you.

As with any form of exercise, first you need to get into some comfortable clothing. Whatever works best for you: sweats, shorts, sport bra, tank top, tee shirt, light pants.

Next establish a regular time of the day to do your workout. This makes it easier to continue the program. Some people like to get up early and do their workout before going to their regular job. For this you'll need about an hour, to do your workout, shower, dress, have a quick breakfast and then get away.

Others would rather do the routine in the evening after the day's work is done. This is riskier, because other activities and social events can jump up and shoot your schedule into small bits and pieces.

Establish your time and try to stick to it.

After that, find the workout records at the end of the book and work out your exercise schedule. Put down the exercises you'll do and the day of the month. After you do each exercise, check it off on your chart.

A chart page will help you to maintain your schedule. As soon as you miss a day that blank space in there will haunt you and help you to get in your workout three to five times a week.

READY, EXERCISE...NO, HOLD IT, WARM UP FIRST

Just a minute. Before you do any form of exercise, you need to warm up. That's next. A warm-up is important for several reasons. First it gets your body moving and working. As you do some small exercises, they help to warm up the body, get the blood circulating faster and your heart beat up to help support your increased activity.

A warm up can help you prevent injury or muscle pulls when you get into your daily exercise routine. A slow warm up will help to stretch ligaments and muscles and give you greater flexibility.

The ideal warm-up is to do each of the following exercises for fifteen to twenty seconds each. Doesn't seem like much but when you're stretching muscles and warming them up, the twenty seconds may seem much longer. This isn't supposed to be a strenuous part of your daily routine.

It's a start, a beginning.

Now, to the first warm-up exercise:

NECK FLEXING

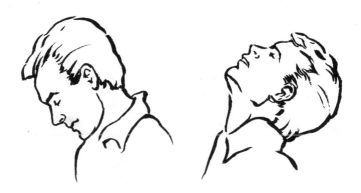

* Standing, hands on hips.

* Drop your chin to your chest as far as possible. Strain to push it down farther. Hold for five slow counts.

* Now slowly lift your head and stare at the ceiling, forcing your head as far toward your back as possible. Strain for five seconds.

* Relax and shake head.

* Repeat exercise five times.

NECK CIRCLES

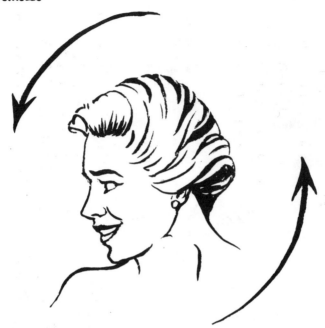

* Stand with hands on wall for balance.

* Lower chin toward your chest, then slowly rotate it to the right forcing it as far back, to each side and front as possible.

* Stress hard with this exercise.

* Rotate five times to the right. Stop and rotate five times to the left. Relax.

ACHILLES, CALF TENDON STRETCHER

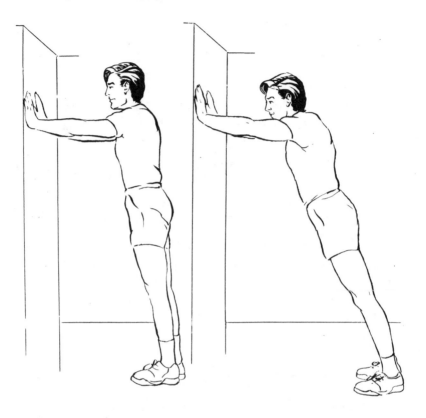

* Stand near a wall. Lean out with arms straight, hands on the wall.

* Gradually work your feet backward until you can feel the tendons stretching and straining in the back of your leg and ankle.

* Keep your feet flat on the floor. Stretch the tendons slightly more by bending your arms a little and leaning farther forward. Hold this stretching for 20 seconds. Then relax.

LEG STRETCHES

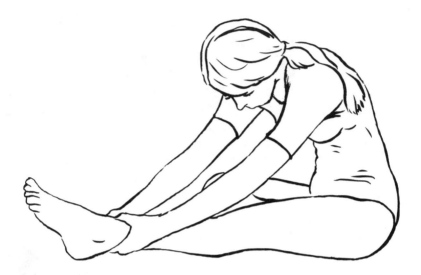

* Sit on your bench or floor. Bend one leg to the side and place one leg straight in front of you.

* Grasp ankle or foot and bend forward at waist as far as you can go stretching back and leg muscles.

* Increase this exercise slowly until you become flexible enough to bring your head closer to your leg.

* Hold this stretching with small increments of forward pressure for 20 seconds. Repeat with alternate leg.

RUNNER'S STRETCH

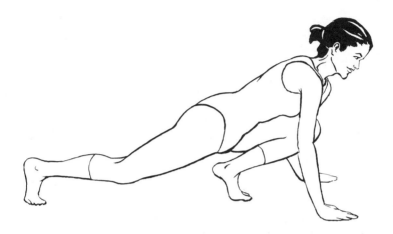

* Squat on the floor and put both hands on floor in front of you.

* Stretch out your right leg behind you as far as you can resting it on your toes. Hold the stretch for ten seconds.

* Return right leg forward and stretch back the left leg the same way.

* Do five reps of the exercise, then relax.

To complete your warm-up, ride a stationary bicycle for five minutes or walk around your yard, or your street for six minutes, then return. Now, you're ready to start your first set of belly flattening exercises.

Three Steps to Flatten Your Belly

Chapter Four
FLATTEN YOUR STOMACH EXERCISES

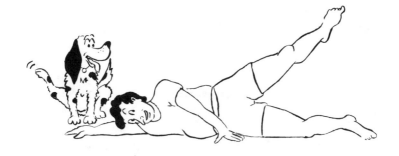

You've done your warm up, now comes the time for your workout on your stomach muscles. These are the obliques both internal and external, the transverse muscles, and the frontal muscles.

To start we have a group of eight stomach flattening exercises for you. As with any new physical activity, you should start this program slowly. We recommend that you begin with four reps of each exercise.

Work through all eight of the exercises this way, remembering to strain the muscles involved at their maximum during the exercise for greatest benefit.

We suggest that you do the four reps the first week, then if you feel at ease and comfortable with that number, to move on to the second developmental level which is an increased number of reps. In the back of the book is a chart for you to use as you get stronger and feel the need for a tougher program.

If you feel that four reps needs to be repeated again for a second week since some of the eight exercises are still hard for you, by all means repeat the four reps. Move on to the next developmental level only when you're pleased with the way you carry out the reps of the entire routine for that day.

#1 ONE ARM, ONE LEG RAISE

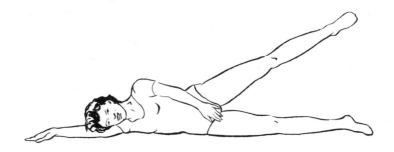

* Lie on a pad with your right arm extended over your head. Rest your head on your arm. Left arm straight, hand at waist.

* Lift your left leg to a 45 degree or greater angle.

* Now raise your left arm to a 45 degree or greater angle and at the same time return your left leg to the start position.

* Return your left arm to original position and at the same time, raise your left leg again.

* Repeat number of reps required, then turn and do the same number on your other side.

#2 SIDE STRETCH LIFTS

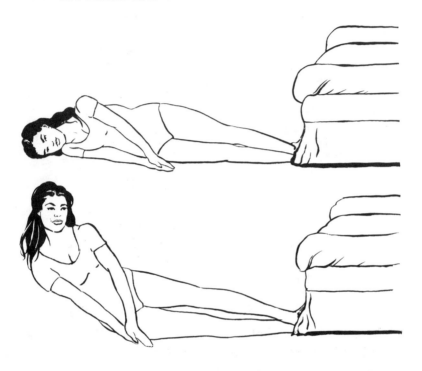

* Lie on your right side with arms in front at your waist. Have someone hold down your feet, or put them under the edge of a piece of heavy furniture.

* Lift your body from the waist up several inches and strain for a few seconds.

* Lower to starting position. Do required number of reps.

* Turn over and repeat sequence on your left side.

#3   CURL-UP TWIST

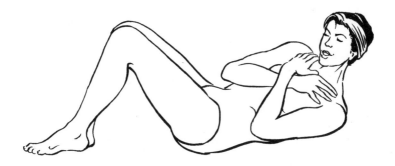

* Lie on your back with knees bent and hands crossed on your chest or behind your neck.

* Curl your head and shoulders off the floor by tightening your abdominal muscles. Keep your back on the floor.

* As you come upward twist to the right and hold for six seconds.

* Return to starting position.

* Repeat curl-up and twist to your left.

* Return to starting position.

* Do required number of reps.

#4   ONE LEG SIDE RAISE

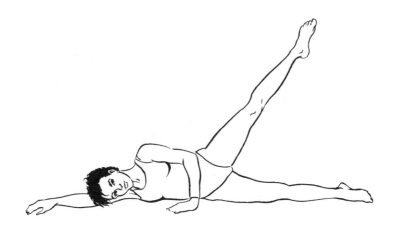

* Lie on your right side, head resting on extended right arm. Left hand on floor at your waist for support.

* Lift your left leg to at 45 degree or more angle.

* Return leg to start position.

* Repeat number of reps.

* Turn over and do on the other side required number of reps.

#5 DOUBLE KNEE SWINGS

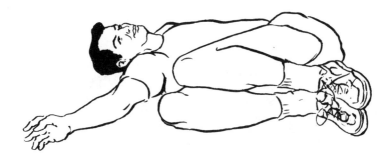

* Lie on your back, arms extended, knees drawn up to chest.

* Keep knees together and swing them to the right until knee touches the floor.

* Return to start position, pause.

* Swing knees to the left until knee touches the floor.

* Return to start position.

* Do required number of reps.

#6   SHOULDER CRUNCH

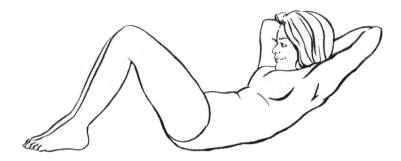

* Lie on the floor, legs bent at a 45 degree angle hands behind head.

* Flexing abdominals, raise head and shoulders off the floor as far as possible.

* Do not lift back off floor.

* Straining, hold position for six seconds.

* Gently lower shoulders and head to floor.

* Repeat required number of reps.

#7 SITTING 'V'

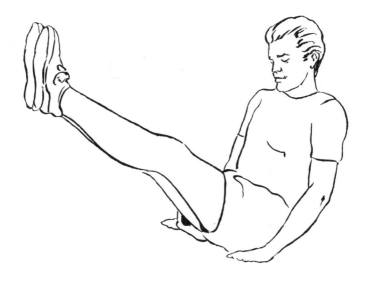

* Sit on the floor with your legs extended, hands beside your hips on the floor.

* Lift your legs off the floor, keeping them together. Tilt your upper body backward until you form a "V." Your back should be slightly rounded.

* Hold the "V" for six seconds.

* Slowly return to start position.

* Repeat required number of reps.

#8   BENT KNEE LEG LIFT

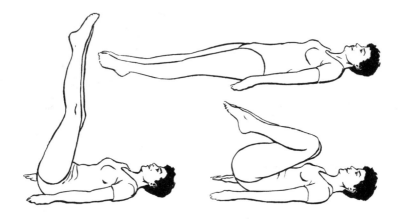

* Lie on back with legs straight out on the floor and arms at your sides.

* Bring both knees hard against your chest, keeping back flat against the floor.

* Lift both legs upward with knees straight so your body forms an "L."

* Return your knees to your chest.

* Return legs flat to the floor.

* Repeat number of required reps.

So, there you have your workout for the day. But you're not done once you finish your reps for exercise #8. Now comes your cool down process.

If you quit exercising cold turkey, you can create problems. Your body has been revved up to some serious exercise, now suddenly you stop, and it doesn't know what to do. You need to cool down gradually, to let your muscles relax and not work so hard. Your heart beat needs to come down slowly to your normal level. Your respiration also will slow down a little at a time.

A sudden stop of exercises after strenuous exercise can cause blood to collect in muscle tissue and veins which can lead to weakness and a sudden dizziness and black spots in front of your eyes.

So, take a few minutes and do these cool down exercises after each workout session.

COOL DOWN EXERCISES

ACHILLES AND CALF STRETCH

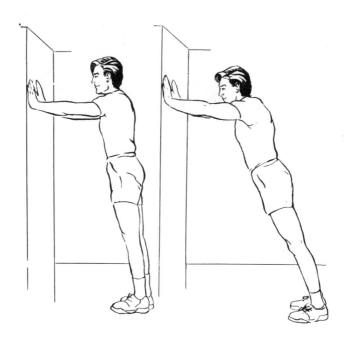

* Stand near a wall. Lean out with arms straight, hands on the wall.

* Gradually work your feet backward until you can feel the tendons stretching and straining in the back of your leg and ankle.

* Keep your feet flat on the floor. Stretch the tendons slightly more by bending your arms a little and leaning farther forward. Hold this stretching for 20 seconds. Then relax.

LIGHT BACK STRETCH

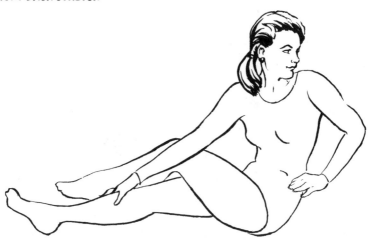

* Sit flat on the floor with legs in front.

* Allow your right leg to stay straight, place your left foot on the floor on the other side of your right knee.

* Hold your straight leg with your right hand. Left hand on your hip.

* Twist upper body to the left as far as possible. Tighten muscles and hold for six seconds.

* Return to start position.

* Repeat with other leg reversing legs, hands and twist.

* Do this exercise three times.

HIGH STRETCH

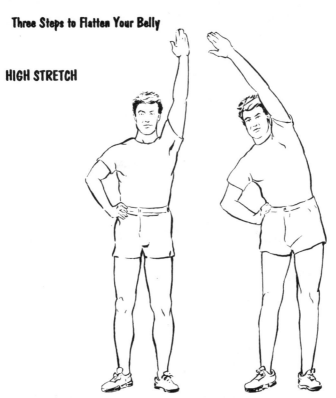

* Stand with feet apart, keep legs straight.

* Place right hand on your right hip, fully extend your left hand over your head.

* Bend slowly to the right. Hold the position for six seconds.

* Change arm positions and bend to the other side and hold for six seconds.

* Repeat this exercise three times.

COOL DOWN WALK

Now do a three minute cool down walk, start fast, then slow down until you are at a leisurely pace by the end of the three minutes. Now hit the showers!

Chapter Five
ALTERNATE EXERCISES

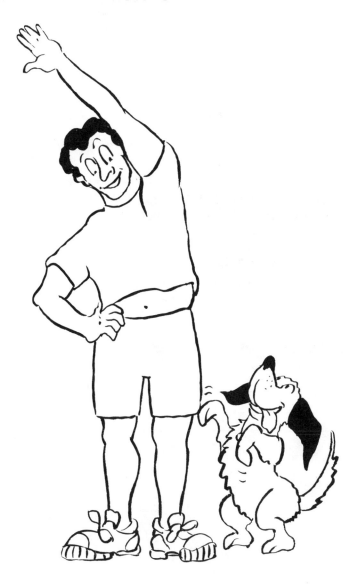

Doing the same eight exercises day after day can get boring. So do yourself a favor. Every so often substitute one of the following exercises for one of the proscribed eight. Or substitute three or four or all eight.

All of these next ten exercises are good workouts for your stomach flattening program. It's just that you can't do eighteen exercises every day and hope to do much of anything else.

When you substitute one exercise for another, circle that exercise's number on your workout chart. You may need to reduce the reps on a new exercise and you may not. If you're at the eight rep step and you get a new exercise, you may want to drop it back to four and work it up to your level on the others.

Or you may be getting in better shape and can pick up the new one at the level of the others, because you're getting leaner and meaner and stronger at the same time.

Here are ten alternate exercises:

#9   DOUBLE LEG SIDE LIFTS

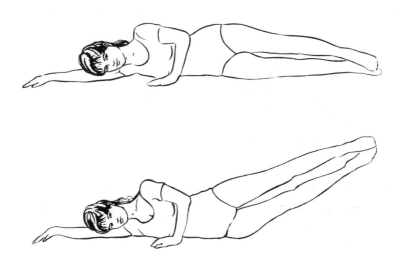

* Lie on your right side, one arm stretched out with your head resting on it. Legs together. Left hand palm down on floor beside your chest.

* Keep legs together and lift them six inches to a foot off the floor. Hold for three seconds.

* Slowly lower legs to start position.

* Repeat doing required number of reps.

* Turn on other side and repeat the exercise doing required number of reps.

#10 LAY DOWN FOOT TO FINGER

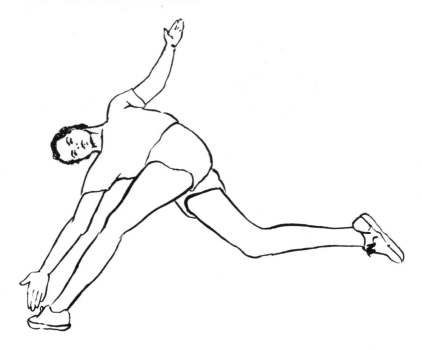

* Lie on your back with your legs together. Push out your arms fully on each side on the floor.

* Lift right leg to vertical.

* Keep knee from bending and swing right leg to the floor to touch your left fingers.

* Return leg to vertical, then lower to floor to start position.

* Do the same exercise with your left leg.

* Repeat for the required number of reps.

#11   RISE UP AND TWIST

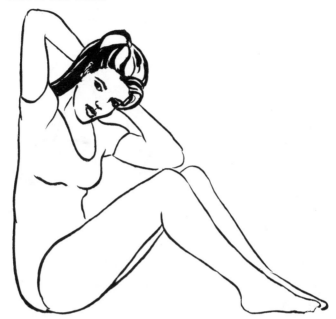

* Lie flat on the floor on your back, bend your knees upward, lock fingers behind your head.

* Gently curl up into a sitting position. First draw your chin toward your chest, then lift your torso upward with stomach muscles. Back should be gently rounded.

* Twist your upper body and touch your right elbow to your right knee.

* Return to starting position.

* Repeat exercise touching left elbow to left knee.

* Do the required number of reps.

(NOTICE: IF THIS EXERCISE HURTS YOUR BACK DO NOT USE IT.)

#12   SLIDE UP AND TWIST

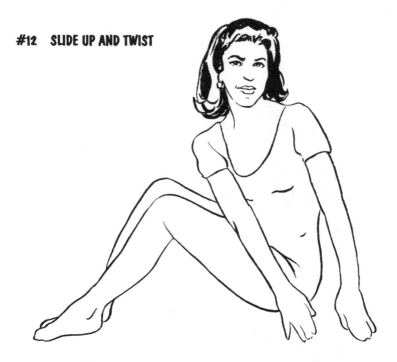

* Lie flat on the floor, legs together, arms stretched down middle of your body.

* Lift your upper body off the floor as a sit up, and at the same time bend up your knees and slide your feet toward your buttocks. Stop at a 45 degree angle. Keep back straight.

* As you curl upward, turn your upper body to the left and touch both hands to the floor on your left.

* Return to starting position.

* Repeat required number of reps alternating sides with the twist.

(NOTICE: IF THIS EXERCISE HURTS YOUR BACK, DON'T USE IT.)

#13   LET DOWN CRUNCH

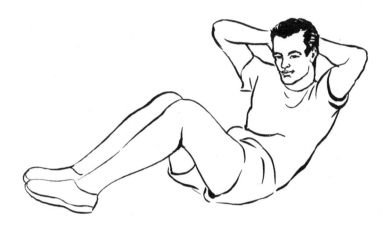

* Sit on the floor and bend your knees up to a 45 degree angle and your hands behind your head.

* Lower slowly your torso backwards to a 45 degree angle. You'll feel your muscles begin to pull.

* Hold for four seconds, then slowly return to start position.

* Repeat the exercise for the required reps.

#14   BENT LEG SIT UPS

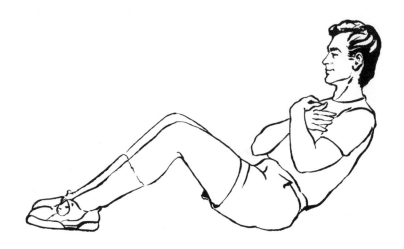

* Lie on your back, legs bent at 45 degree angle, arms lax at your sides.

* Pull down chin toward your chest then lift your torso up in classic sit-up. Back should be slightly rounded.

* Return to start position.

* Repeat exercise the required number of reps.

(NOTICE: IF THIS EXERCISE HURTS YOUR BACK, DON'T USE IT.)

#15   BENT KNEE SINGLE LEG LIFT

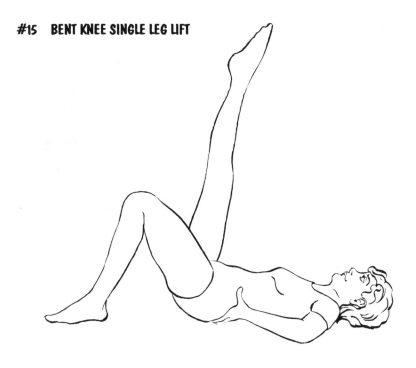

* Lie on your back, left leg bent upward at 45 degrees. Right leg flat on floor. Hands on your hips.

* Lift your right leg straight up to vertical. Keep the small of your back firmly against the floor.

* Bring down your right leg to the floor.

* Repeat required number of reps.

* Now reverse legs and do the exercise the required number of reps lifting your left leg.

#16   FLOOR BICYCLING

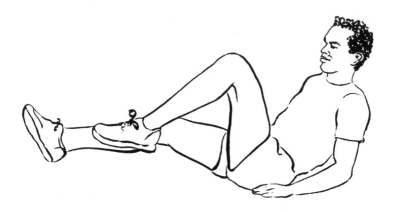

* Sit on the pad with your hands by your hips and your legs extended.

* Lift one leg up and pull toward your chest. Lean back a little and keep your back slightly rounded.

* Lift your other leg off the floor and simulate a bicycle motion with both legs but don't touch the floor.

* Each stroke with your left leg is one rep. Do three times the required reps.

#17   CURL TOE TOUCHES

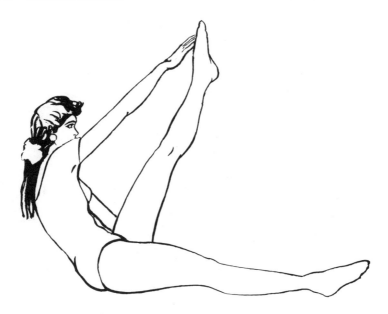

* Lie on floor with legs stretched out fully and arms near your sides.

* Curl your body forward in near sit up position and at the same time lift your left leg and lift right arm and touch your left toes.

* Return to start position.

* Curl up again using other hand to touch your other toe and return to start position.

* Repeat required number of reps.

(NOTICE: IF THIS EXERCISE HURTS YOUR BACK, DON'T USE IT)

#18   V SEAT WALKING

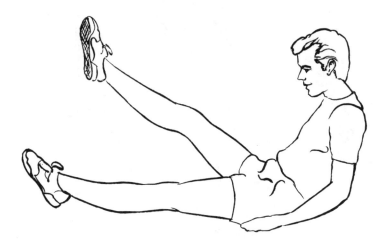

* Sit on floor with legs extended and your hands on the floor near your hips.

* Lift your legs off the floor to a 45 degree angle and lean torso slightly to the rear for balance. Back is slightly rounded.

* Move your legs up and down in opposite directions as if walking without touching the floor.

* Each right leg up is one rep. Do three times required reps for this exercise.

VARIETY OR EXTRA WORK EXERCISES

These are the other exercises you can work into your program. Some you may like, some not. Some will be harder than others. Be sure you have two or three extremely hard ones in your eight part program. The hard ones mean you need more work on those muscles.

Substitute exercises in your workout chart whenever you wish, but give at least a three week try on one exercise before you move to another one. Enjoy.

Three Steps to Flatten Your Belly

CHAPTER SIX
BIG BONUS POINTS!

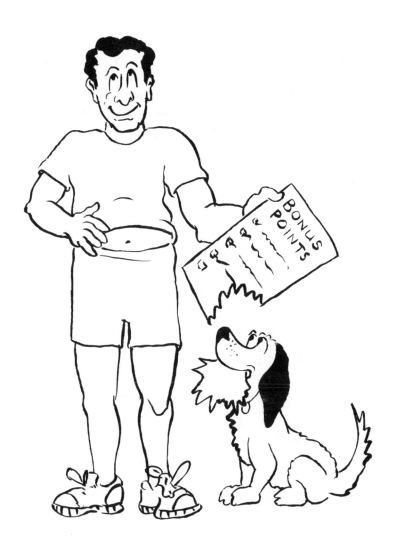

Okay, so far so good. You have your exercise program, you're starting to work at it five times a week, step two and three are coming up. You still wonder if there's more you can do on those odd moments during the day when you aren't working or playing or in your regular exercise program.

Fact is, there is.

Here are a few "off line" exercises that you can do. Some of them you can do sitting at a computer or desk. Some you can do while you're walking down the hall or in your office with the door closed.

Again these exercises are aimed at your stomach muscles, and at trimming your waistline. Which is about the same thing. So think of these as that "extra credit" work you need to tie down that "A" grade in your course, "Belly Flattening 101." Go ahead, try them and enjoy.

**EXTRA CREDIT
#19 LIFT THE TABLE**

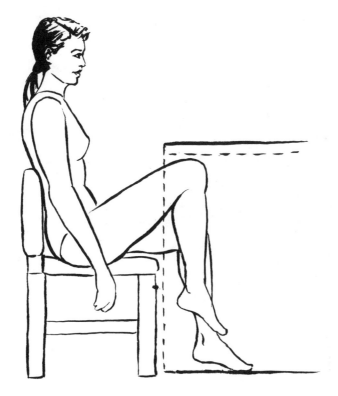

* Sit at a table, desk, or a restaurant booth.

* Lift one leg so knee touches underside of table.

* Press upward as if to lift the table. Keep up the pressure for ten seconds.

* Let that knee down and do the same with the other knee.

* Repeat alternating legs until both have done the exercise three times.

EXTRA CREDIT
#20   EXTENDED LEG DESK LIFT

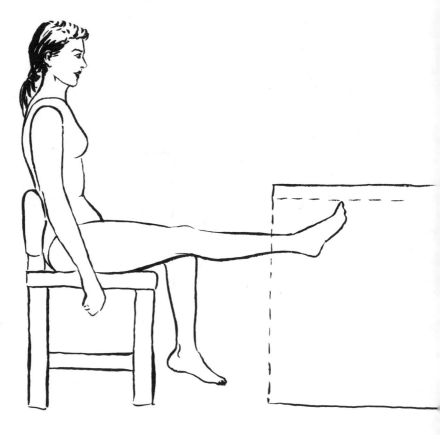

* Push upward with your toe putting pressure on the desk. Hold for ten seconds.

* Return that foot to the floor.

* Do the same with the other foot holding pressure for ten seconds.

* Now repeat the exercise until each leg has done the exercise three times.

EXTRA CREDIT
#21   CHAIR LEAN BACK

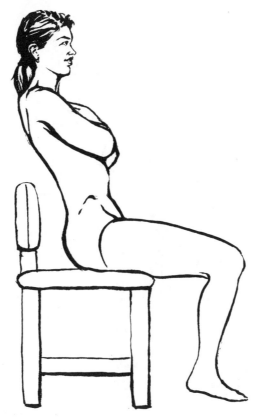

* Sit on very front edge of chair or bench. Arms crossed, feet together on floor. Lean back slowly until your back almost touches the chair. If you don't feel a strain on your stomach muscles, move out farther on the front edge of chair.

* Hold position for ten seconds.

* Slowly sit forward.

* Repeat this exercise six times.

EXTRA CREDIT
#22   STANDING STRETCH

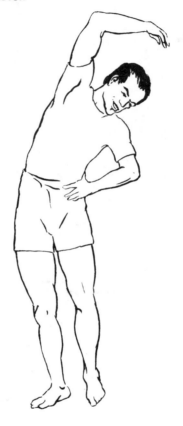

* Stand with feet a foot apart, right hand on hip, left arm extended over head.

* Stretch your torso slowly to the right, stretching your left hand over your head to the right. Stretch as far as you can five times.

* Change hands and to the same thing to the left.

* Repeat the left-right exercises three times.

EXTRA CREDIT
#23   LEAN BACK, LIFT KNEES

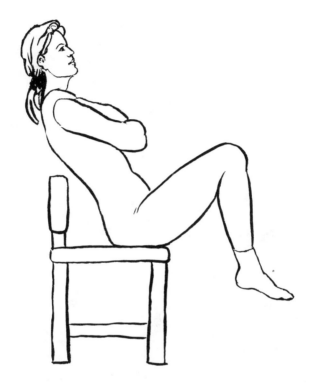

* Sit on very front edge of a chair. Both feet resting on the floor, arms folded on chest.

* Lean back slowly without touching back of chair. At the same time, lift your knees off the floor. Stress muscles. Hold for a five count.

* Return to start position.

* Repeat ten times.

EXTRA CREDIT
#24   STANDING TRUNK TURNER

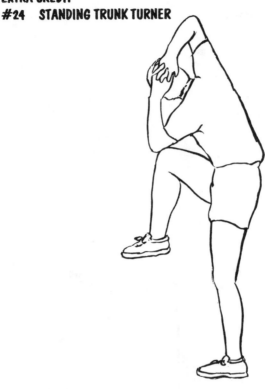

* Stand with feet a foot apart, and hands clasped behind head. Elbows pushed to rear as far as possible.

* Lift your right knee as high as possible directly in front of you.

* At the same time, bend and reach down with your left elbow to touch your right knee.

* Return to start position.

* Do the exercise again with right elbow touching left knee and return to start.

* Do six reps of this exercise.

Remember, these are not a part of your regular work-out. They are for those minutes during the day you could do a few exercises and not interfere with your regular work routine.

If you do substitute some of these for your eight major exercises, be sure to do the number of reps that your correct progress level advises.

Three Steps to Flatten Your Belly

STEP TWO

BURNING OFF THE FAT

Three Steps to Flatten Your Belly

Chapter Seven
THE OLD AEROBIC TRICK

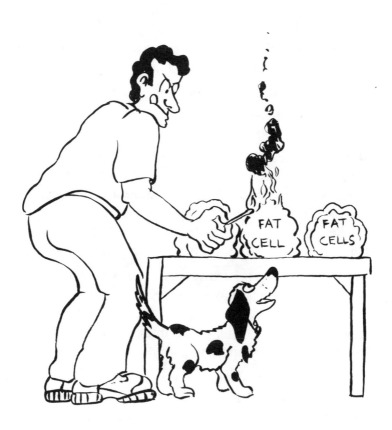

Now, you have a good start on your exercise program. You're faithfully working those selected exercises three to five times a week. You're starting to feel the muscles pull in and tighten.

Great!

We move ahead to the Second Step in the program, burning off some of that ugly fat. As we talked about before, the abdominal muscle exercises are not designed to burn off excess fat. They are to tone and strengthen the stomach muscles so you can have that hard, flat belly when the excess fat is gone.

Now we come down to the de-fatting process. It is fat, don't be shy about the word. You'll be hearing a lot about it in the next two steps.

This whole idea of losing weight comes down to one simple fact. You simply must burn off more calories every day than you stuff into your mouth. Nothing to it, right? Wrong. Look at the hundreds of diets on the market, at the thousands of weight loss programs, pills, drinks, machines, lotions and wraps.

Human nature makes it easy to eat, tough to exercise, and much harder to make a commitment to yourself that you will lose weight and keep it off and establish a new approach to eating your three meals a day—the low-fat healthy approach.

Most doctors say that the best way to burn off calories is to get your body in motion, then keep it in motion. Experts say that if you walk, run or swim or do any active sport for 20 minutes without stopping, you will have done a good deed for your heart by strengthening it.

Use that time zone and then keep going for another ten to twenty minutes and you are now doing a good turn for your waistline. The longer you walk, run, bike, swim or do any other aerobic exercising without stopping, the more calories you'll burn off and the better chance you'll have to lose weight.

Remember, this is step two for flattening your stomach. One was exercising those stomach muscles. This is step two where you concentrate on burning off the fat cells. From there we leap into how to learn how to establish new eating habits so you take in fewer fat calories, so you have fewer yet to burn off.

Most people stay relatively close to their body's needs on intake and burning off of calories during their daily lives. For Example if you eat food that inputs 2,200 calories during a 24 hour period, and your body during its normal course of activities burns off 2,200 calories that same day, you won't lose or gain any weight.

Let's say you love good cooking, and big meals, that you take a fancy to another beer just before bed, or you love those chocolate candies, and as that continues you are now taking in 2,400 calories, but still only burning off 2,200 during the day. That means you gained 200 calories that day.

No big deal? Not those 200 calories. Nutritionists tells us that one pound of fat on the body can be produced by 3,500 calories.

Say you eat that extra 200 calories each day for a month. That means you have taken in 6,000 calories more than you burned off. If you keep doing that for six months, your figure will now show a nice roly-poly gain in weight of more than ten pounds. Over a year you would be a rounded 140 instead of the svelte 120 you started out as on New Year's eve.

Look at it the other way. Say you start your aerobic workouts and do them every day. Make it a habit like putting on your shoes and brushing your teeth.

In the process you keep your diet the same at 2,200. But in that time you have learned how to eat low-fat meals and you watch sweets and cut down on those late night beers and low and behold you are now taking in only 2,100 calories and thriving on it.

You are also doing your aerobics and you're burning off another extra 100 calories a day. The result is that you are now taking in and burning off 200 calories more than you eat. Simple arithmetic means that in six months of this you can slice ten pounds of ugly fat off your body. Men will lose most of this from their bellies and waists. Women will lose in about equal amounts from thighs, hips and belly.

Hey, we're getting there.

Now those five times a week abdominal exercises you still do, will begin to show a harder, firmer stomach with three or four pounds less fat to conceal the real you.

Aerobic exercises simply burn off calories efficiently, gradually, and with no hard strain. When you go on a long walk, for example, your heart speeds up, your blood vessels expand to carry more blood and oxygen to your cells, your breathing quickens and gets deeper to supply more oxygen your body needs, and in the process you start burning off more calories.

Some specialists say that when you do good aerobic exercising of any type you will burn off about 100 calories in nine or ten minutes, depending on the degree of exertion. That multiplied by a thirty minute hike means you've burned off 300 calories.

This is the reason there is a step two. Your stomach muscle exercises are not designed to burn off fat. They are to tone up your muscles. We need them.

Weight lifting, the hard iron workouts, are designed to add muscle to your body. They do not burn off excess fat. That you still have to do with aerobic exercising and a good low-fat eating system.

HOW MUCH BURN-OFF, HOW FAST?

Which is the best of the aerobic exercises? Just how many calories does walking burn, compared to a man running a six minute mile for the same time frame? These estimates are worked out on the basis of a person weighing 150 pounds. For each fifteen pounds more than this, add 10% to the calorie burning figure. For each 15 pounds less than this, take off 10%.

For example a man who weighs 165 pounds would be burning off 165 calories each 15 minutes when he walked upstairs.

A woman weighing 120 pounds would burn off 120 calories per 15 minute workout walking upstairs.

CALORIE BURN-OFF CHART

Exercise	Calories burned in 15 minutes
Walking, 3 miles per hour	65
Walking, 4 miles per hour	100
Walking up stairs	150
Walking up hills	125
Aerobic Dancing	100
Bicycling, 6 miles per hour	70
Bicycling, 10 miles per hour	105
Stationary Exercise Bike, moderate	70
Running, 12 minutes per mile	143
Running, 8 minutes per mile	215
Running, 6 minutes per mile	260
Rowing Machine, fast	110
Nordic Track Machine	150
Swimming, crawl stroke	145
Stair climber machine	155
Treadmill, moderate speed	120

SO HOW DO WE START?

The first step is to decide which type of aerobic exercising you want to do. When we say aerobic most people think of the sleek, happy, jumping dance aerobic classes you see on TV advertisements and in movies.

Aerobic Dancing   Yes, aerobic dancing is one of the good ways to use in this Step Two of burning off the fat. A word about a word. Aerobic means simply: "a method of physical conditioning designed to improve respiratory and circulatory functions through continuous exercises." Aerobic exercising isn't limited only to aerobic dancing, but that certainly is a popular one.

How can you do this? There are many video tapes on the market you can get and do a half-hour to 45 minute session in your living room or your family room. These tapes are usually good, but they come at various levels of expertise, so get one that matches your physical ability and your level of competence at aerobic dancing.

You can join a gym and take their dance classes, or you can join a class of aerobic dancing in a hall or even at your work place. Some employers are now offering exercise rooms and aerobic classes for their workers, knowing that a healthier person makes a happier and more efficient worker in almost any type of employment.

Aerobic dancing can get extremely strenuous. Check with your doctor to be sure what level of aerobics you should do. Try to stay somewhere close to the type recommended for your age group. If you're twenty, you'll want to get in a vigorous young group.

If you're in your forties or fifties, search around to find an aerobic class that caters to your age group. These days many YMCAs and YWCAs have aerobic classes aimed at those older age groups.

Don't overdo it. As with the tummy flattening exercises, take it easy as you start out. If you can find an easy aerobics video, this is a good way to start, since you can go at your own pace and quit when it gets too much.

At home alone? Try to find a neighbor who is also interested in some exercise and invite that person over for a regular workout. It's always more fun exercising with someone else, then too, you'll be more likely to keep up a program if you have two or three or four neighbors dropping in three to five times a week for your exercise program.

Walking   Yes, check the chart above. Walking is a great way to get in your aerobic workout for the day. The great thing about walking for your aerobics is that you can do it by yourself, you can go anytime of day or night that you want to, you can vary the time of day from day to day, you can go faster or slower as you wish. You can also go farther or shorter, and you can pick out the route. Nothing to say you can't walk on the beach in the summertime and enjoy the sights and sounds of the surf and sand and those marvelous new bikini swim suits.

"Can walking really be beneficial? It seems so simple."

Exactly. Walking is simple, natural and it's been around for a long, long time. It's bound to stay here. Why?

Many people say that walking is the simplest and safest way to get in your aerobic conditioning work. Because it puts a stress on your lungs, walkers are not as likely to smoke cigarettes as more inactive people.

Walking can also help you to relieve the stress of the day. It can do a lot to improve your mood and clear up your thinking.

Important for us in this program is that walking can help you take off weight and keep it off. Some even think that walkers become more concerned with their health so they build up good nutritional habits. Whether due to the better eating habits or better circulation, walking is thought to slow down osteoporosis a problem for many older women.

What about the person who says that walking is fine, but why not speed up the benefits by running. Fine, give running a shot. I've done a marathon, a run of 26 miles 285 yards. It's a long ways. I spent over six months and 1200 practice miles getting ready for the big day.

I made it, without a record, and I admit that I started out too fast and had to walk several times. But I made it. After the thrill of the marathon, I kept running, but I tapered off then to a four mile run a day. It seemed so short and done so quickly.

Two months later my left knee told me it was tired of running. The knee's cartilage was simply wearing thin on some of the vital places it was needed in there. I stopped running.

Much later, I began walking. The walking actually strengthened the knee so it no longer gave me any trouble.

Why did running do me in? Running lifts the whole body off the ground and your foot, ankle, knee and hip take the pressure as you land and stride forward. Each time your foot hits the ground or pavement, it hits with a force of three times your body weight.

A basketball player going up for a lay up or jamb or jump shot can come back to the maple floor with the force of seven times his weight. That's one reason many basketball players have foot and knee problems.

Walking doesn't put these tremendous strains on the body's joints because there's not jolt.

Most walkers use the heel-to-toe method of walking. You hit on your heel and roll forward to the ball of the foot and push off with the toe. Simple, shock free and easy.

Some folks who know tell us that every day in this nation of ours, more than 65 million people take part in some form of exercise, sports or aerobic training. Guess what their favorite form of workout is? Right....walking.

It's simple, inexpensive, can be done anytime, anywhere, and it can be done alone or with somebody. No waiting for a tee time, no trying to get a tennis court, no looking for a hoop to use for your round ball practice, and no trouble with not getting the team together to practice. Walking is not a team sport. Hooray!

How's your heart? Over the past 30 years, heart attacks have tapered off a little. This is due to many factors, including fewer smokers and more exercise.

No test have been done on a scientific basis to prove

that aerobic walking can reduce your chances of having a heart attack, but most professionals in the health field, say the evidence is undeniable. Aerobic walking will not only help you trim the fat off that belly of yours, but at the same time will be a big factor in helping your heart to gain in strength and in function.

Not a bad partnership, I'd say.

One small way you can test this. It's called your resting heart rate. Right now, before you dig into this program, take time out and record your resting heart rate.

Not hard. Oh, the best place to take your pulse is on the carotid artery in your neck. It's larger, stronger has more blood pumping through it than your wrist, and is easier to find and maintain.

So, sit down in your favorite chair and do nothing for five minutes. TV is approved, but no humor show that will have you breaking up every 20 seconds. At the end of the five minutes take your pulse.

The easiest way to do this is to use a stop watch or sweep second hand or stop watch feature on a sport digital watch. Get your forefinger on your carotid and wait for a steady pulse. You should be able to feel it easily. Don't press so hard you cut off the flow. Pick up the count and stay with the pulsations for ten, then look at your watch. Check the timer at an even ten second point, 20, 30, etc. Count each heart beat for 15 seconds. Say you get 20 beats. Now multiply that 20 by four, to get the number of beats per minute. You have an 80.

Most adults have a resting heart rate from 50 to 90. Generally the lower your resting heart rate, the better your physical condition.

Now, write this figure and the date in your permanent health record, or on the Workout Record section in this book or on the flyleaf or back cover. Just don't lose it. We'll be looking back at that figure again in three months to see how much improved your resting heart rate is.

Shoes   A lot is made in some quarters about using "walking" shoes in your aerobic walking. True walking shoes are hard to find, terribly expensive and not all that much different from running shoes.

True walking shoes often are made of leather rather than nylon and tend to trap your foot sweat. Running shoes have good heels and soles that will absorb the shock of hard landings on the average runner.

This makes them work just fine for walking. Your impact won't be as hard on walking, and the running models offer better absorption of the forces so they aren't transferred to your ankle and knee joints.

The fact that most running shoes offer much better ventilation is another plus for the walker.

Sweat   All feet sweat. When you walk they sweat more and even though the running shoes have ventilation panels, you still need good socks to absorb most of that moisture. Cotton socks are the most absorbent and will do a good job. Whether you wear the low socks or higher ones is up to you.

Oh, don't plan on walking in the same pair of shoes

every day. You should alternate your shoes. Just the way they made you do in the army with your combat boots, remember? Same idea. Your shoes will have a chance to dry out completely, and your feet will get the benefit of a different pair of shoes. They might look identical, but no two shoes are exactly alike. The foot print will be different inside the shoe due to differences in construction and materials. Change here every other day is good.

Foot care Most people, experts figure about 90 percent of the men, women and children in our land, have feet good enough to walk for an hour or two a day with no problems.

The more you walk, the more you'll realize that it pays to take care of your feet. With good cotton socks, some walkers like to wear two pair of socks, a thicker pair and a thinner one, your feet shouldn't get blisters.

If you get blisters, you're doing something wrong. Maybe you're pushing off too hard, or your shoes don't fit right or your socks are bunching up and causing too much pressure. Take care of your feet. You're going to need them for a long time.

You might want to dust some antifungal powder into your socks before your walk. Can't hurt. If you do get a blister, break it with a sterilized needle as soon as you get home.

It's always a good idea to wash your feet after a workout on any kind of aerobic foot work, dancing, stair climber, walking, running, Nordic Track, or treadmill, even an exercise bike.

Try the old shock treatment. Use a bucket and fill it with cold water. Then run hot water in your bath tub. Lower the bucket of cold water into the tub and soak your feet in the cold water first for a minute, then plunge your feet into the hot water. This alternately restricts and expands the blood flow in your feet.

Do this six times, then dry off your feet. They'll feel delightful. This treatment helps to tone your tissues, muscles and ligaments. Besides, it feels just great.

Swimming   Swimming is one of the favorite aerobic exercises for some people. Swimming is a more difficult workout than walking since it exercises more muscles of your body, especially your arms and upper body.

For a time, some people thought that swimming couldn't be an aerobic fat burner because of the temperature of the water. The colder than body temperature water tends to increase a thin layer of body fat just under the skin to protect the body from the cold.

This is true, however the increased body fat is slight and you will more than compensate for that and burn off a lot of excess fat in other locations of your body with any kind of sustained long distance aerobic swimming for 30 minutes or more.

The secret to swimming as an aerobic exercise is to get good at it. Develop a powerful, rhythmic crawl stroke, that puts your breathing on automatic pilot so you don't have to think about it. You hit the end of the pool, make your speed turn or a slow turn and you're moving again.

Those who feel totally at ease in the water, who say that swimming distances is as easy and natural for them as walking, will find the most benefit. They will get a restful and relaxation benefit as well.

The fat burning is our main concern here. Pace yourself. A hard swimming workout will burn more calories than the same time walking. Actually the rate is more than double. If you swim for a half hour without a break, you'll be burning off more calories than on an hour and a half walk.

Keep track of your swimming on your workout record listing either distance or time, but be consistent. Use the same stroke and pace for each day so you'll have a realistic comparison.

Stair Climber   These machines are comparatively new when put up against the longevity of walking and swimming. Since most of them can be adjusted for difficulty, they can be an extremely good aerobic exercise.

If you aren't familiar with the stair climber, they consist of a pair of long pedal like levers and an upright frame that you hold on to. The levers go up and down as you walk and are loaded to give more or less resistance when you step up and down on them.

These machines come in all sorts, styles, sizes and sophistication. Some are electronically monitored so you can program in flat and even walking, up hill and down, and a slower and faster pace. These are not strength machines. They are designed for the long haul of aerobic exercising and therein lies their greatest value.

Utilize a stair climber the way you would any other exercise program. If not used to the machines test yourself on them until you find a comfortable and slightly difficult level. Work at that level until you find you need to increase the resistance or the time.

Remember that we're pointing toward at least a 30 minute aerobic workout. This is your main fat burning program. This is the one that will let you see results in your battle of the bulge.

Cost of these machines may be a factor. There are some for less than a hundred dollars and others that run to six hundred. If you're buying one, test it completely first. Many people get experience on stair climber machines in a gym, find out the type they want and even the brand, then get a somewhat smaller and lighter and less expensive version of the same machine for their home workout room.

Keep a record on your workout report of the level and the time spent on the machine. Your purpose here is to do these exercises five times a week.

Stationary Exercise Bike   The indoor bike is a mainstay of many people's aerobic exercise workout. The bikes themselves are relatively low cost, most can be set for varying levels of difficulty, and you can do your exercises in any room in your home from your bedroom to the living room to the family room.

Some people read books while they do their 30 to 45 minute workout. Others watch TV or listen to the radio or records or books on tape.

If you live in a neighborhood where you'd rather not go outside to do your three mile walk, the exercise bike can take care of your aerobic workout nicely. They are also handy to replace your outdoor run or walk when it's raining cats and poodles or the temperature has bottomed out somewhere near Nome, Alaska and the Huskies are barking on your rear doorstep.

Since the exercise bike can be programmed for stress and you can control the time precisely, many people these days are turning back to the bike for their workouts. Be sure to keep a record and put down the speed and difficulty as well as the time involved.

Treadmill   Most of the things said about the convenience and safety and comfort of the exercise bike also applies to the treadmill. One big difference is the cost. Some of these treadmills can be quite costly if you go for the ones with all of the built in electronic programming and various speeds and up and down hill workouts.

The treadmill should not be used by anyone who has a poor sense of balance or who is unsteady on his or her feet.

Treadmills have gained a surge in acceptance in big city areas where a running man can often draw a policeman's attention as well as stray dogs and muggers. They are also extremely handy when winter weather rolls around and you need to get in your 45 minutes of workout so you don't have a blank spot on your workout record book.

Keep track of your aerobic workouts on the record sheet in back of the book.

Nordic Track   The Nordic Track is typical of the many stationary ski exercise machines now on the market. Here you're working indoors with all of the benefits.

The ski machine does more for your workout because it gives you the aerobic exercising and at the same time gives your arms and shoulders additional work.

These cross country type ski machines come in a variety of makes and models. Get one that will do what you want it to do and keep in your price range.

THE AEROBIC WORKOUT

So, there you have the aerobic workout. This is the one that's going to chop the fat off your body. Work at it regularly, with enthusiasm. Walking remains the simplest, cheapest and one of the best aerobic workouts. Running and fast swimming probably are the exercises that will do you the most good in the quickest time investment. The ski machines and treadmills and stair climbers will be the most expensive ways to burn off that ugly fat.

Whichever one you decide to do, make up your mind that you're in for the long haul. Set yourself a goal, and to get there be sure that you do your 30 to 45 minute workout five times a week. Figure out how many calories you want to burn off. Say a brisk walk for an hour should burn off about 400 calories. If you run at a six-minute a mile pace for half an hour, you'll burn off 520 calories.

Whichever aerobic activity you choose, make it fun.

And remember that you can change from time to time. You can walk for a month or two, switch over to the stationary bike for two months, then do swimming for a time. Just be sure to keep up your calorie burning time that you need.

Three Steps to Flatten Your Belly

STEP THREE

LOW-FAT EATING

Three Steps to Flatten Your Belly

Chapter Eight
CHANGING YOUR EATING HABITS

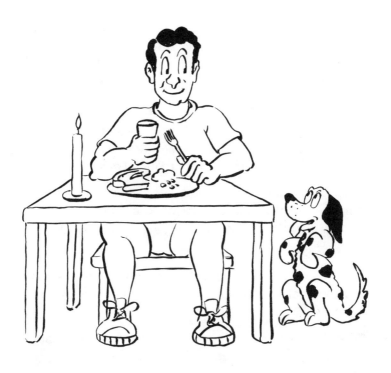

We homo sapiens are creatures of habit. Absolutely true. We get habitual about everything we do. We say, "Oh, my schedule was thrown off and nothing went right." or that "I always do it that way."

Eating is another habit we have. Most of us are the products of the hard-working American laboring force where three square meals a day were required. If you have a farm background you ate breakfast, dinner and supper because you needed those three high energy meals a day.

Some health experts say we would be much better off if we ate two lighter meals a day, with an eye to satisfying our body's nutritional needs, rather than to satisfy our appetites.

However, those three meals a day are a ritual we won't break for another century at least, so we need to learn how to plan our eating habits so we can be eating healthy and cut down on our fat caloric intake.

When we talked about total calories consumed before, we didn't break it down into the various types of calories. Basically there are three, fat, carbohydrates and protein.

The biggest problem with more calories comes when a great deal of those calories are eaten in the form of fat.

The simplest way to lose weight is to take into your system less fat than you burn off every day. The way the body stores energy is in fat cells. It can store it and store it until you weigh much more than you should or want to.

By controlling the input of fat calories in your diet, you can literally ignore the number of non-fat calories that you eat every day.

The amount of fat calories you eat each day determines almost entirely whether you will gain or lose weight.

Just what do we mean by foods with fat calories? What are these foods? Here are a few of them that you'll recognize at once:

Whole milk and cream, potato chips, sour cream, regular cheeses of all kinds, ice cream, regular mayonnaise, regular salad dressing, tuna fish in oil, gravies, ground beef, milk shakes, doughnuts, regular cakes, pies, puddings, any fried foods, all French fried foods.

You say stop, stop, stop. That paragraph contains the best foods in the Western world. In there are all of your favorites. There is no chance that you can simply cut out all the foods with high fat content and remain mobile, reasonable or sane.

Good, we're not saying you have to cut out all of those foods. Hold your judgement for a minute and let's look at the rest of this low-fat eating idea before you pitch out the diamond ring with the silver polish.

Let's take a check on how much fat you include in your diet every day. Almost nobody can give a figure for the number of grams of fat he or she eats every day. Most people who are concerned worry about total calories and not grams of fat.

Most of us have some realization that most dairy products are loaded with fat, as well as doughnuts, and cakes and pies and of course chocolate fudge. But we don't realize that a lot of snack foods, most fast food, and most deserts and even juicy steaks are high in grams of fat as well.

Let me give you a teaser. How would you like to eat all of the non-fat calories a day that you want to? Most of us who watch our eating habits would say great. What's the catch? You can eat all the calories you want to, if you keep your fat intake down in a realistic level. Another way to say that is if you keep your grams of fat down to the level that your body needs.

You do need fat for a healthy diet, no one is arguing that. But what you don't need is our American high-fat eating habits.

Let's go a step farther and say if you maintain our suggested low-fat intake, you can forget about counting calories, and you will lose weight on this three step plan.

Something else to think about. A new study by the U.S. Department of Agriculture shows that nine out of ten Americans do not get an adequate amount of chromium in their daily food intake. This could be the result of most people not eating enough foods that contain trace elements of chromium. Another reason might be that much chromium is lost in processing and cooking of those foods that have the chromium. Then again, the soil where the foods are grown could be heavy or short on chromium and that lack could show up in the foods.

Now on the market to help solve this problem is a product called Chromium Picolinate that is said to help you to lose body fat while maintaining vital muscle tissue.

Chromium occurs naturally in small amounts in foods including brewer's yeast, black pepper, lobster and liver.

NEVER COUNT CALORIES AGAIN.

Yes, that's right. All you have to do is this: For women, keep your fat intake between 22 and 38 grams of fat a day. For men the figures are between 28 and 60 grams a day. Men get a higher gram level because most men have a higher activity level than most women. Adjust your intake accordingly. Men, if you sit behind a desk all day, drive to work, and use a power driven lawn mower at home, you don't need such a high fat intake either.

Now, think this way. You won't be counting calories, but you now need to count up your fat gram total. Think what foods have those big grams of fat totals, and which ones don't.

Right away you'll come up with the realization that most fruits and vegetables have almost no grams of fat. Lots of bulk and vitamins and carbos, but almost no fat. Naturally we'll be pushing for more fruits and vegetables in your diet.

Here are some other foods with extremely low fat content. Dried fruits of all kinds qualify, almost all vegetables from asparagus down to zucchini, alphabetically speaking.

Most of the breads are low in fat, just so you don't soak them with piles of butter. These include regular large and small loaves of sliced bread, bagels, English muffins, hard dinner rolls, tortillas and pita bread.

You see, already we're coming up with a lot of foods that you like that will keep you away from the dreaded fat gram gorilla.

More foods low in fat include almost all dry and cooked breakfast cereals. If you put a tablespoon of butter in your cooked white rice, you'll defeat the goal of a low-fat breakfast.

Dry cereal? Yes, but you can use milk on it. Skim milk or 1% milk will work just as well, once you adjust to the slightly different taste.

Crackers qualify here as low-fat, everything from grahams to saltines and rice cakes and pretzels.

We didn't mention grains when we talked about vegetables. These also are low-fat or no fat: corn, rice, wheat, oats, and grain products such as macaroni, noodles and spaghetti.

Also on the list of low or no fat foods are the starchy ones such as potatoes, yams, all kinds of dry beans and peas.

So, what this low-fat eating program is doing is giving you a large variety of foods to select from, but limiting the high fat foods to the minimum. Come on, you can do that. You do want to get rid of that bulge around your tummy and those thunder thighs and wasteland waist? Good. Let's move on.

COMMON SENSE EATING

You can switch your eating habits to low-fat without all that much fuss. Take some basics: pasteurized milk. High in fat content. Instead use skim milk or 1% milk. You'll get used to the slightly different taste in a rush. Here are a few more common sense alternatives to high fat food that you will soon get used to and wonder why you ever ate any other way:

. Ice Cream....go to sherbets or low-fat desserts. There are also low-fat ice creams and ice milks on the market these days that are comparatively low in fat.

. Regular salad dressing....use lite or low-fat types.

. Ground beef..30% fat......switch to ground turkey, or 15% fat hamburger.

. 2 eggs and bacon....use three egg whites, pitch out the yolks. Add boiled and then pan-fried potatoes lightly salted with onions mixed in last few cooking minutes.

. Tuna fish canned in oil....use water pack instead.

. Fried fish....broil, bake or poach the same fresh fish.

. Vegetables in cheese sauce...steam vegetables and serve with spices, herbs, lemon juice.

. New York sharp cheddar cheese....find low-fat cheeses.

. Candy bars, M&M snacks... go instead with fresh fruit or dried fruit.

. German chocolate cake.... instead try angel food cake.

. Buttered toast......instead of margarine or butter use non-fat jam or jelly. No cause to worry about the fat calories here.

SOUND TOO DIFFICULT?

You say all this gram counting is too much trouble? Hey, you're two thirds of the way to a slimmer, harder you. You're doing your stomach exercises, you're working on fat burning aerobics, now all you have to do is watch the old fat intake.

It isn't that hard at all. Hey, what about a can of tomato soup for lunch? Throw in a can of milk and you still only have two grams of fat. Say you had five saltine crackers with the soup and a piece of toast and jam. That's another gram of fat for the toast and two for the crackers. No don't put margarine or butter on the toast, just with the jam which has sugar and calories but no fat. A cup of coffee or tea or a big drink of ice water. Five, maybe six grams of fat at the most for your whole breakfast. Not bad when you can eat from 30 to 60 grams a day.

Let's back up and have breakfast: Juice, half an apple, a cup of dry cereal with 1% milk, half a slice of toast and some marmalade. How many grams of fat? Maybe three grams of fat even with the low-fat milk.

That wasn't so hard.

Now for a low-fat dinner. So far today you've had about ten grams of fat. That means you can have 20 more if you're a woman, 50 more if you're a man. What's for dinner?

How about three pieces of roasted chicken, six ounces, with the skin peeled off. Dark meat about 2.5 grams of fat an ounce. White meat is 1 gram of fat an ounce. Say the chicken cost you 12 grams. Throw one medium sized potato in the oven during the chicken roasting, heat up a can of green beans, make a tossed green salad with lettuce, onions, radishes, sliced cabbage and some croutons along with half a tomato, add black coffee or tea and you have a good little dinner. The fat count? Chicken, 12 grams, potato with salt and spices and a touch of milk to mash it, 1 gram, the beans 1 gram a cup, the salad with two teaspoons of low-fat salad dressing goes for 3 grams, and the slice of dark bread and jam is another gram. The total cost in grams: 18 or 19 grams. Now come on, wasn't that a good dinner?

What was your total for the day? 19 grams for dinner, breakfast went for four and lunch at six. That's 29 grams of fat for the day. Top it off with a mixed fruit salad made from half an orange, half an apple and a banana, all cut into half inch squares and tossed for your snack while you watch TV. Throw in a half a small snack sized bag of microwave popcorn for another 2 grams.

Your day's intake of fat counts up to only 31 grams, since the fruit, the green beans and the crackers have almost no fat content.

See what I mean?

Look at the side panel on a can from your cupboard. Whether it's beans or soup or tuna fish, there will be a chart listing the amount of food values, including one for fat, shown in grams.

Get used to looking at these little charts. They'll come in handy in helping you to plan out interesting, appetizing, healthful meals that will keep you low on the old fat content.

Fruits and vegetables can fill you up in a rush and give you no fats at all. Cereals, legumes, beans, breads, pasta (with a reasonable sauce) also carry almost no fat penalty.

When you buy meat, buy the leanest cuts you can find. Ask your butcher to give you some service. Even in the big supermarkets there's a butcher on call to cut what you want. Have him trim off all the fat and suggest the leanest cuts for your low-fat diet. He'll help you.

OTHERS IN THE HOUSE?

You say all this is fine for one person, but you have a spouse and three growing kids in the family. They always want something to eat as well.

A healthy, low-fat diet will be just as good for the kids and your ultimate other as it is for you. What's not to like? You can have all sorts of pastas, potatoes a dozen different ways, fish broiled, lean cuts of meat, your own thin broiled hamburgers (so the fat runs out of them) with all sorts of good lettuce, onions and other nutritious additives in the "mom's secret sauce."

Yes, you will need to do a little planning before you go shopping. That's a good way to get some variety into your meals. You might come up short and need to rush down to the supermarket another time during the week, but it all will be worth it.

It won't happen all at once. Binges will break out. (A Carl's Junior double western bacon cheeseburger runs 63 grams of fat. But most burgers cost you about 20 to 40 grams of fat.) On the long pull, you'll have you and your family on a healthier diet, you'll be changing their eating habits for the better.

SOME FOODS TO AVOID

Generally you can eat almost anything, but there are some heavy fat penalties to pay if you do. Here is a list of foods that you should look at carefully and decide how your fat total is for the day before you buy or order one of these.

Food	Grams Fat
Tuna packed in oil	15
Smoked bratwurst	21
Bearnaise sauce	68
Pepperoni pizza	32
1 cup pecan halves	72
1 hot dog	18
Sausage, eggs, hash browns	34
Frozen fried chicken dinner	29
Frozen chicken/noodles dinner	72
Arby's Cashew Chicken Salad	37
Baskin-Robbins 2 scoops ice cream	28
Burger King Croissant Sausage Sandwich	40
Carl's Jr. Super Star Hamburger	53
Dairy Queen's Ultimate Burger	47

Dunkin' Donuts Glazed Chocolate Ring	21
Haagen-Daz 4 oz. Butter Pecan Ice Cream	24
Jack in the Box Grilled Sourdough Burger	50
KFC Extra Crispy Thigh	30
Long John Silver's 3 pieces fried fish and french fries	53
McDonald's Quarter Pounder With Cheese	28
Quincy's Steakhouse 13 oz. T-bone Steak	159
Red Lobster Ribeye Steak, 12 oz.	82
Roy Rogers RR Bar Burger	39
Winchell's Donuts Apple Fritter	37

Pig out days? Yes, there will be some, especially with teenagers. But by eating two meals a day at home during school days, they'll learn healthy eating habits from your example. Fresh, frozen and canned vegetables and fresh fruits can't be over emphasized.

Just you? Much easier. Give it a try, if you don't like it you can always go back to wearing those big cover-up swim suits once the beach season arrives.

Just kidding. You can stick to a low-fat program. You can do it. For a jump starter, here are three days sample menus for you. See what you think:

THREE DAY LOW-FAT MENU:

Day 1: Breakfast: six-ounce juice of your choice; hot cereal: oatmeal w/raisins, brown sugar, 1% milk or skim milk on cereal; coffee, tea or ice water.

Fat Grams: 3

Lunch: water-pack tuna, 2 ounces for sandwich, 1 teaspoon mayonnaise, $1/_4$ cup chopped onion, 2 teaspoons pickle relish, 2 slices whole-wheat bread for sandwich; carrot and celery sticks; one medium orange; 8 ounces lemonade, ice water or coffee.

Fat Grams: 6

Dinner: 6 ounces baked turkey breast; fresh boiled broccoli; $1/_2$ baked acorn squash with 1 teaspoon margarine, one teaspoon brown sugar; fresh fruit salad: $1/_2$ apple, $1/_2$ pear, $1/_2$ banana; 1 heated dinner roll and jelly or jam; 8 ounces milk, coffee, tea or ice water

Fat Grams: 17 to 19

Total Fat Grams for Day 1: 30 to 32

Day 2: Breakfast: 1 grapefruit juiced with pulp; 1 cup dry cereal, 1% milk, sugar; 1 whole-grain toast, jam; milk, coffee or tea.

Fat Grams: 4

Lunch: 1 poached egg; 1 slice toast, jam; $1/_2$ pear or apple; milk, coffee or tea.

Fat Grams: 8

Dinner: 4 ounces of fish fillet baked in foil; carrots, potatoes, green beans; 1 French hard dinner roll; 1 cup sherbet desert; milk, coffee or tea.

Grams Fat: 7 to 10

Total Fat Grams for Day 2: 22 to 24

Day Three: Breakfast: 6 ounces fruit juice: 2 slices French Toast with jam; 2 slices bacon; $\frac{1}{2}$ banana; milk, coffee or tea.

Grams Fat: 22

Lunch: $\frac{1}{2}$ cup minestrone soup; 5 Saltine Crackers & jam; $\frac{1}{2}$ pear; milk, coffee or tea

Grams Fat: 7

Dinner: large serving spaghetti, meatless spaghetti sauce; 1 slice whole grain-toast with garlic spread; tossed green salad, vinegar dressing; slice cherry pie; milk, coffee or tea.

Grams Fat: 19

Total Grams Fat for Day 3: 48

Now, you get the idea. Check on the list of various foods and the amount of fat content they have per serving in the next chapter to plan your meals. After a while you'll know that a pancake is worth 10 grams right off the bat. Butter can add another 3 to 5 and don't even think about syrup. (Just kidding!)

Yes, it will take a little thought right away. You might have cornflakes the first week for breakfast, but then you'll start thinking about other things that will keep your fat count down and it will become a challenge and soon a game that will be fun to play.

And......you'll be able to watch that belt line shrink and that stomach tighten and the fat cells scream in surrender and fade away into the night.

Go now and eat high fat content foods seldom more.

Chapter Nine
COUNTING THOSE GRAMS OF FAT

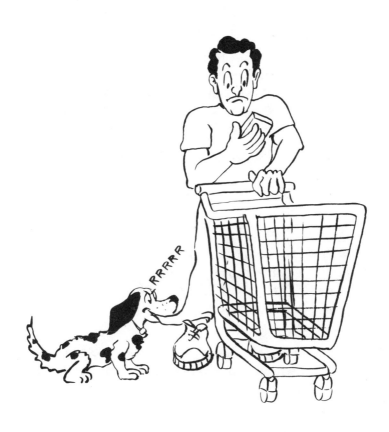

RRRRR

Just how do you know how many grams of fat are in the food you eat? The best way is to take a look on the can or carton in the supermarket when you shop. After May 1994 all food products must have their contents of fat and calories plainly spelled out somewhere on the product.

Every product designated as a food must have this information on it. If the product is too small to have it printed there, there must be a phone number where the purchaser can call and get the information.

But, what about the fast food place and a fancy restaurant? No such charts are listed beside each dish on the menu. No wonder when a nice T-bone steak can cost you 160 grams of fat, not counting all the sauces and side dishes.

With restaurants, you have to figure the odds. You know some basics: any fried food is going to be ten times as high in grams of fat as the same product broiled or boiled. So be careful of fried foods, especially deep fried foods.

That lowly potato has only a trace of fat when raw or boiled. But turn it into French fries and it draws from 12 to 18 grams of fat per serving. One ounce of Pringle's Butter and Herbs potato chips runs you 13 grams of fat.

In the following chart, I'm going to show you a list of some of the representative foods and how they rate with fat content. No attempt is made to separate saturated from unsaturated fat.

On fruits I'll show you two or three with the note that there is about the same amount of fat in all fresh fruit, which is almost zero.

The same samples will be given for a variety of foods and products that you can take a clue from.

If you want to get more serious, there are paper back books on the market made up of nothing but fat and calory counts for every imaginable food and a run down on many of the popular fast food chains with their products detailed. Some of these fat counter books run to over 500 pages.

Here then is an abbreviated and representative list of foods and their fat content:

FOOD CHART SHOWING FAT GRAMS PER SERVING

Note: The following foods are listed in category alphabetically. They are listed by food group, not as "apple" but apple is shown under fruit. Some products are listed by themselves, but all are in categories such as: bread, cakes, eggs, margarine, pasta.

Since many of us are also interested in the calorie count on food, I'll also list the calories for each serving.

Food	Serving	Fat Grams	Cals
Bacon:			
Armour Star, cooked	1 slice	3	38
Oscar Mayer, cooked	1 slice	3	35
Nathan's Beef Bacon	3 slices	7	100
Beef:			
Tenderloin	3 oz.	12	208
Top round	3 oz.	8	170
Top sirloin, fried	3 oz.	19	277

Food	Serving	Fat Grams	Cals
Beer:			
Schlitz	12 oz.	0	145
Miller Lite	12 oz.	0	96
Bread:			
Weight Watcher's			
Cinnamon Raisin	1 slice	Trace	60
Pepperidge Farms	1 slice	3	90
Wonder, Wheat	1 slice	1	70
Light Oatmeal	1 slice	0	45
Pita, whole wheat, 1 pocket	1 oz.	1	80
Roman Meal	1 slice	1	68
French bread	1 slice	1	100
Butter:			
Cabot	1 tsp.	4	35
Land O'Lakes	1 tsp	4	35
Land O'Lakes Whip	1 tsp	3	25
Cake Mixes:			
Angel food	$1/12$ cake	0	150
Banana cake	$1/12$ cake	11	250
Carrot cake	$1/12$ cake	15	232
Chocolate & Chocolate frosting	$1/8$ cake	17	300
Date quick bread	$1/12$ loaf	2	160
Lemon cake, frosting	$1/8$ cake	17	300
Crumb coffeecake	$1/6$ cake	7	230
Candy:			
Almond Joy	1.76 oz.	14	250
Butterfinger	2.1 oz.	12	280
Hershey Bar w/Almonds	1.45 oz.	14	240

Food	Serving	Fat Grams	Cals
Lifesavers	1 candy	0	40
M & M Peanuts	1.7 oz.	13	250
Mr. GoodBar	1.7 oz.	19	290
Gum drops	1 oz.	0	100
Cereals: with ½ cup 1% milk:			
Alpha Bits	1 cup	1.5	212
100 % Bran	⅓ cup	3.5	170
Apple Raisin Crisp	⅔ cup	1.5	230
Bran Flakes	1 oz.	2.5	200
Ralston Rice Chex	1 cup	1.5	194
Froot Loops	1 cup	2.5	210
Corn flakes	1 cup	1.5	210
Quaker Life	⅔ cup	3.5	200
Quaker 100% Natural	¼ cup	7.5	227
Cream of Wheat	1 oz.	2.5	208
Instant oatmeal	1 cup	3.5	245
Cheese:			
Blue cheese	1 oz.	8	100
Brie	1 oz.	8	95
Armour Cheddar	1 oz.	9	110
Bristol Gold Lite	1 oz.	4	70
Colby	1 oz.	9	110
Edam	1 oz.	8	100
Kraft Gouda	1 oz.	9	110
Monterey Jack	1 oz.	9	110
Swiss	1 oz.	8	110
Chicken:			
Breast quarters w/skin	1 oz.	2	42

Food	Serving	Fat Grams	Cals
Breast quarters skinless	1 oz.	Trace	31
Leg quarters w/skin	1 oz.	4	49
Dark meat batter dip	5.9 oz.	31	497
Dark meat, roasted	3.5 oz.	16	256
Banquet Fried Chicken	6.4 oz.	19	330
Swanson Fried Chicken	4.5 oz.	20	360
Chili:			
Chef Boyardee Chili Con Carne w/ Beans	7 oz.	20	340
Dennison's Chili w/Beans	7.5 oz.	19	300
Van Camp's Chili w/Beans	1 cup	23	352
Health Valley Vegetarian	5 oz.	3	160
Potato Chips:			
Eagle Chips	1 oz.	10	150
Kelly's Rippled	1 oz.	9	150
Lance Rippled	1 oz.	13	160
Pringle's Chips	1 oz.	13	170
Weight Watchers Barbecue	1 oz.	6	140
Coffee:			
Instant regular, black	6 oz.	0	4
Regular brewed, black	6 oz.	0	4
Cookies, Ready To Eat:			
Nabisco Raisin Oatmeal	1	3	70
Angel Bars	1	5	74
Lance Apple Oatmeal	1.65 oz.	7	190
Anisette Toast Jumbo	1	1	109
Chips Ahoy Choc-Walnut	1	6	100
Nutra/Balance Choc Chip	2 oz.	14	260

Food	Serving	Fat Grams	Cals
Lance Choc-0-Mint	1.25 oz.	10	180
Heath Valley Apple Spice	3	Trace	75
Tastykake Fudge Bar	1	8	240
Frookie Ginger Spice	1	2	45
Sunshine Lemon Coolers	2	2	60
Cottage Cheese:			
Borden 5% Dry Curd	1/2 cup	1	80
Knudsen 2%	4 oz.	2	100
Land O'Lakes	4 oz.	5	120
Weight Watchers 1%	1/2 cup	1	90
Crackers:			
Nabisco Cracked Wheat	4	4	70
Goya Butter Crackers	1	1	40
Cheese crackers w/P butter	1.4 oz.	11	210
Cheez-it	12	4	70
Dark Rye Crisp Bread	1	Trace	26
Nabisco Escort	3	4	70
Keebler Garlic Melba toast	2	Trace	25
Saltines	2	1	25
Frozen Dinners:			
Armour Classic Chick/Noodles	11 oz.	73	230
Armour Lite Chicken Ala King	11 oz.	7	290
Banquet Chicken Nuggets	6 oz.	16	340
Budget Gourmet Chic. Caccit.	1 pkg.	27	470
Budget Gourmet Lite Pot Roast	1 pkg.	8	210
Le Menu Beef Stroganoff	10 oz.	24	430
Le Menu Lite Glazed Chicken	10 oz.	3	230
Lean Cuisine Fillet Fish	10 oz.	5	210

Food	Serving	Fat Grams	Cals
Swanson Chicken Nuggets	9 oz.	23	470
Weight Watchers Baked Fish	7 oz.	4	150
Doughnuts:			
Tastykake Chocolate Dipped	1	10	181
Earth Grains Devil's Food	1	21	330
Powdered sugar minis	1	3	58
Tastykake Fudge Iced	1	21	350
Glazed donuts	1	13	235
Eggs:			
Fried with margarine	1	7	91
Hard boiled	1	5	77
Scrambled	1	7	101
Egg white only	1	0	17
One egg yolk poached	1	5	59
Egg Beaters (substitute)	$1/4$ cup	0	25
Scramblers (substitute)	3.5 oz.	5	105
Fish:			
Smelt	6 oz.	6	212
Red snapper	6 oz.	3	217
Microwave tuna sandwich	1	6	200
Rainbow trout broiled	3 oz.	4	129
Canned tuna in water	3 oz.	2	90
Canned tuna in oil	3 oz.	15	200
S&W canned tuna in water	3 oz.	1.5 oz.	90
Orange ruffy baked	3 oz.	1	75
Sea bass, broiled	3 oz.	2	105
Groton's Frozen Scrod	1 pkg.	18	320
Van Kamp's Frozen Fillets	1	10	180

Food	Serving	Fat Grams	Cals
Mrs. Paul's Fish Cakes	2	7	190
Microwave Fish Sandwich	1	15	280
Fruit:			
Fresh apple	1	Trace	81
Fresh grapefruit	$1/2$	0	40
Dry, pitted prunes	$1/4$ cup	1	140
Fresh orange	1	Trace	69
Fresh pear	1	1	100
Fresh pineapple	1 cup	1	90
Canned mixed fruit	$1/2$ cup	0	90

* Most fresh fruits have almost no grams of fat. Canned fruit have little more, but the sugar content raises the level of the calorie count.

Food	Serving	Fat Grams	Cals
French Toast:			
Home-made with egg, milk	1 slice	7	155
Take-out, with butter	1 slice	9	180
Aunt Jemima Cinnamon Swirls	3 oz.	4	71
Weight Watchers French Toast	2 slices	5	160
Gelatin:			
Royal Apple	$1/2$ cup	0	80
Jell-O Black Raspberry	$1/2$ cup	Trace	81
Cherry w/Nutrasweet	$1/2$ cup	Trace	8
Diamond Crystal Orange, sugar-free	$1/2$ cup	Trace	9
Gravy: (canned)			
Franco-American Beef	2 oz.	1	25
Franco-American Pork	2 oz.	3	40
Pepperidge Farm Beef	2 oz.	2.5	65

Food	Serving	Fat Grams	Cals
Ham:			
Armour Star Boneless	1 oz.	2	41
Hansel 'n Gretel Deluxe	1 oz.	1	31
Krakus Polish cooked	1 oz.	3	65
Oscar Mayer Cracked Black	1 oz.	Trace	24
Russer Lill' Salt cooked	1 oz.	1	30
Canned extra lean	1 oz.	2	41
Hamburger:			
Double patty w/bun	1 reg.	28	544
Double patty, all fixings	1 reg.	32	576
Double patty, all fixings	1 large	44	706
Single patty, w/bun	1 reg.	12	275
Single patty, bun, cheese	1 reg.	15	320
Single patty, all fixings.	1 large	48	745
Triple patty, all fixings	1 large	51	769
Hot Dogs:			
Chicken:			
Health Valley	1	8	96
Weaver	1	10	115
Turkey:			
Bil Mar Cheese Franks	1	9	109
Louis Rich	1	9	103
Mr. Turkey Franks	1	11	132
Wampler Longacre	1	31	102
Beef:			
Armour Star Jumbo	1	18	170
Hebrew National	1	15	160
Oscar Mayer Bun Lengths	1	17	186

Food	Serving	Fat Grams	Cals
Oscar Mayer Wieners Little	1	3	28
Ice Cream, Ice Deserts.			
Bresler's All Flavors Ice	3.5 oz.	0	120
Bresler's Ice Cream	3.5 oz.	12	230
Edy's light Almond Praline	4 oz.	5	140
Sealtest Butter Crunch	½ cup	9	160
Lady Borden Butter Pecan	½ cup	12	180
Haagen-Daz Chocolate	4 oz.	17	270
Weight Watchers Ice Milk	½ cup	4	120
Ben & Jerry's Chocolate Fudge	4 oz.	16	280
Good Humor Chocolate Malt	3 oz.	13	187
Weight Watchers Treat Bar	2.75 oz.	0	90
Breyers Coffee Ice Cream	½ cup	8	150
Mocha Mix Dutch Chocolate	3.5 oz.	12	210
Land O'Lakes Fruit Sherbet	4 oz.	2	130
Wyler's Fruit Punch Slush	4 oz.	0	140
Ben & Jerry's Health Bar	4 oz.	17	300
Jell-O Orange Bars	1	Trace	42
Borden Orange Sherbet	½ cup	1	110
Jams, Jellies:			
Smucker's Fruit Spreads	1 tsp	0	16
Pritikin Fruit Spreads	1 tsp	0	14
White House Apple Butter	1 oz.	0	50
Bama Grape Jelly	2 tsp	0	25
Apple Jelly	3.5 oz.	0	259
Strawberry Jam	3.5 oz.	0	234
Plum Jam	3.5 oz.	0	241

No jams, jellies, fruit preserves, etc. have any grams of fat. The only difference is in the calorie content.

Food	Serving	Fat Grams	Cals
Luncheon Cold Cuts:			
Armour Bologna Beef	1 oz.	8	90
Carl Buddig Pastrami	1 oz.	2	40
Hansel 'N Gretel Healthy			
Deli Bologna Beef & Pork	1 oz.	2	41
Oscar Mayer Bologna	1 slice	8	90
Oscar Mayer Honey Loaf	1 slice	1	35
Weight Watchers Bologna	1 slice	1	18
Hard Pork Salami	1 slice	4	41
Summer Sausage Thuringer	1 oz.	8	98
Margarine:			
Fleischmann's Diet	1 tbsp	6	50
Mazola Diet	1 tbsp	6	50
Parkay Diet Soft	1 tbsp	6	50
Smart Beat	1 tbsp	3	25
Regular Stick:			
Blue Bonnet	1 tbsp	11	100
Fleischmann's	1 tbsp	11	100
Land O'Lakes	1 tbsp	4	35
Mazola	1 tbsp	11	100
Parkay	1 tbsp	11	100
Soft Tub:			
Blue Bonnet	1 tbsp	11	100
Fleischmann's	1 tbsp	11	100
Land O'Lakes Tub	1 tbsp	4	35
Parkway Soft	1 tbsp	11	100
Promise	1 tbsp	10	90
Parkay Whipped	1 tbsp	7	70

Food	Serving	Fat Grams	Cals
Mayonnaise:			
Low Calorie:			
Best Foods Cholesterol Free	1 tbsp	5	50
Best Foods Light	1 tbsp	5	50
Kraft Free	1 tbsp	0	12
Kraft Light	1 tbsp	5	50
Smart Beat Corn Oil	1 tbsp	4	40
Regular:			
Best Foods Real	1 tbsp	11	100
Hellmann's Real	1 tbsp	11	100
Kraft Real	1 tbsp	12	100
Sandwich Spread	1 tbsp	5	60
Mexican Food Frozen:			
Banquet Chimichanga	9.5 oz.	21	480
Banquet Enchilada Cheese	11 oz.	9	340
El Charrito Burrito Grande	6 oz.	16	430
Enchilada Cheese Dinner	14 oz.	24	570
Corn tortillas	2	1	95
Healthy Choice Enchiladas	13 oz.	5	350
Healthy Choice Fajitas	7 oz.	4	210
Lean Cuisine Enchanadas	10 oz.	9	290
Patio Enchilada Beef Dinner	13 oz.	24	520
Patio Fiesta Dinner	12 oz.	20	460
Van De Kamp's Beef Burrito	5	9	320
Van De Kamp's Mexican Classics			
Chicken Suiza w/Rice, Beans	15 oz.	20	550
Enchilada Suiza Chicken	5.5 oz.	10	220
Weight Watchers Fajitas	7 oz.	5	210

Food	Serving	Fat Grams	Cals
Taco shells	1	2	50
Muffins:			
Frozen:			
Sara Lee Apple Oat Bran	1	6	190
Health Valley Banana Free	1	Trace	130
Sara Lee Blueberry	1	8	200
Sara Lee Blueberry Free	1	0	120
Pepperidge Cinnamon Swirl	1	6	190
Sara Lee Golden Corn	1	13	240
Health Valley Oat Bran	1	4	140
Muffin Box Mix:			
Arrowhead Blue Corn	1	4	110
Duncan Hines Bran, Honey	1	4	120
Duncan Hines Cran-nut	1	8	200
Duncan Hines Wild Blueberry	1	3	110
Milk:			
Evaporated	1/2 cup	10	170
Evaporated Skim	1/2 cup	0	100
Carnation dry milk	8 oz.	Trace	90
1% milk	1/2 cup	1.5	51
2% milk	1/2 cup	2.5	60
Buttermilk	1/2 cup	2	60
Whole Milk regular	1/2 cup	4	75
Skim Milk	1/2 cup	Trace	45
Nuts:			
Cashews, peanuts	1 oz.	12	170
Planters Mixed, Salted	1 oz.	15	170
Guy's Tasty Mix	1 oz.	7	130

Food	Serving	Fat Grams	Cals
Dry roasted w/peanuts	1 oz.	15	169
Planters' Almonds	1 oz.	15	170
Black Walnuts	1 oz.	17	180
English Walnut halves	1 oz.	20	190
Cashews	1 oz.	14	170
Cashews dry roasted	1 oz.	13	163
Filberts	1 oz.	19	191
Peanuts dry roasted	1 oz.	14	170
Peanut butter	2 tbsp	17	200
Pecans	1 oz.	20	190
Cooking Oil:			
Crisco	1 tbsp	14	120
Planter's Popcorn Oil	1 tbsp	13	120
Puritan	1 tbsp	14	120
Wesson Corn	1 tbsp	14	120
Smart Beat	1 tbsp	14	120
Wesson Vegetable	1 tbsp	14	120
Crisco Solid	1 tbsp	12	110
Wesson Shortening	1 tbsp	12	100
Oriental Foods Frozen:			
Benihana Lites Chicken	9 oz.	4	270
Birds Eye Stir Fry Veges.	1/2 cup	Trace	36
Birds Eye Chow Mein	1/2 cup	4	89
Chung King Walnut Chicken	13 oz.	5	310
Chung King Egg Rolls Shrimp	3.6 oz.	6	200
La Choy Pork Egg Roll	3 oz.	5	150
Take Out:			
Chicken teriyaki	3/4 cup	27	399

Food	Serving	Fat Grams	Cals
Chop suey with pork	1 cup	24	425
Pancakes and Waffles:			
From Mixes Made At Home:			
Hungry Jack Blueberry	3 4-inch	15	320
Aunt Jemima Buckwheat	3 4-inch	8	230
Hungry Jack Buttermilk	3 4-inch	11	240
Hungry Jack Packets	3 4-inch	3	180
Arrowhead Griddle Lite	½ cup	3	260
Estee Pancake Mix	3 3-inch	0	100
Pancakes with butter, syrup	3 4-inch	14	519
Pasta			

* Most pastas are 1 gram of fat per 2 oz. The differential here is what is put in the pasta or on it. Calories for plain pasta range from 160 per 2 oz. to 210.

Food	Serving	Fat Grams	Cals
Dry pasta, all types	2 oz.	1	210
Pasta dinners, frozen:			
Banquet entree primavera	7 oz.	3	140
Banquet Macaroni & Cheese	7 oz.	11	260
Budget Gourmet Stroganoff	1 pkg	12	290
Budget Gourmet Cheese Manicotti	1 pkg	25	430
Dining Light Fettucini	9 oz.	12	290
Green Giant Cheese Tortellini	1 pkg	9	260
Healthy Choice Fettucini	8.5 oz.	4	240
Kid Cuisine Macaroni, Franks	9 oz.	15	360
Le Menu Light Tortellini	8 oz.	8	250
Lean Cuisine Rigatoni, Meat	10 oz.	10	260
Morton Macaroni & Cheese	6.5 oz.	14	290
Swanson Spaghetti Meat Balls	13 oz.	18	490
Weight Watchers Manicotti	10 oz.	8	260

Food	**Serving**	**Fat Grams**	**Cals**
Pickles:			

* All cucumber pickles have either 0 grams of fat or a trace.

Pie:			
Frozen:			
Banquet Apple	1 slice	11	250
Sara Lee Apple	1 slice	12	280
Mrs. Smith's Apple Natural	1 slice	22	420
Banquet Banana	1 slice	10	180
Mrs. Smith's Blueberry	1 slice	17	380
Banquet Lemon	1 slice	9	170
Banquet Pumpkin	1 slice	8	200
Baked Ready to Eat:			
Apple	1 slice	18	405
Creme	1 slice	23	455
Lemon meringue	1 slice	14	355
Pizza:			
Frozen:			
Celeste Deluxe	8 oz. slice	32	600
Fox Deluxe Sausage	1/2 pizza	13	260
Jeno's 4 Pack Cheese	1 pizza	8	160
Jeno's Crisp Sausage	1/2 pizza	16	300
Pappalo's French Pepperoni	1 pizza	20	410
Totino's Bacon Party	1/2 pizza	20	370
Totino's Mexican Style	1/2 pizza	21	380
Weight Watcher's Cheese	7 oz.	7	300
Popcorn:			
Jiffy Pop Microwave Butter	4 cups	7	140
Newman's Microwave Light	3 cups	3	90

Food	Serving	Fat Grams	Cals
Redenbacher Gourmet Original	3 cups	4	80
Pillsbury Microwave Butter	3 cups	13	210
Ultra Slim-Fast Lite	1/2 oz.	2	60
Weight Watcher's Ready Eat	.7 oz.	3	90

Salad Dressing:
Ready To Use:

Food	Serving	Fat Grams	Cals
Catalina	1 tbsp	1	15
Diamond Crystal Blue Cheese	1 tbsp	1	20
Kraft Bacon & Tomato	1 tbsp	7	70
Kraft Free Catalina Nonfat	1 tbsp	0	20
Ott's Italian Chef	1 tbsp	9	80
Newman's Olive & Vinegar	1 tbsp	9	80
Seven Seas Free Ranch Nonfat	1 tbsp	0	16

Ready To Use Lite:

Food	Serving	Fat Grams	Cals
Estee Blue Cheese	1 tbsp	Trace	8
Herb Magic Vinaigrette	1 tbsp	0	6
Kraft French	1 tbsp	1	20
Magic Mountain Blue Cheese	1 tbsp	Trace	5
S&W Italian No Oil	1 tbsp	0	2
Ultra Slim-Fast	1 tbsp	Trace	6
Weight Watcher's Russian	1 tbsp	5	50

Sausage:

Food	Serving	Fat Grams	Cals
Oscar Mayer Bratwurst Smoked	2.7 oz.	21	237
Perdue Turkey Patties	1.3 oz.	4	61
Armour Country Sausage	1 oz.	11	110
Hebrew National Knockwurst	3 oz.	25	260
Oscar Mayer Polish	2.7 oz.	20	229
Armour Link Pork Sausage	1 oz.	11	110

Food	Serving	Fat Grams	Cals
Perdue Sweet Italian Turkey	2 oz.	6	94

Soda Drinks:

* All but four of the popular soft drinks now on the market have no fat grams at all. Of the four that do, two are root beer, one a ginger ale and the other a wild berry. Calories vary but go from a low of a trace in diet drinks to 190. Most are about 75 or 80 calories. No big worry about fat grams from soft drinks.

Turkey:

Fresh:

Food	Serving	Fat Grams	Cals
Louis Rich Breast	1 oz.	2	50
Perdue Breast Fillets	1 oz.	Trace	28
Louis Rich Breast Steaks	1 oz.	Trace	40
Perdue Fresh Drumsticks	1 oz.	2	36
Bill Mar Ground Turkey	3 oz.	12	163
Louis Rich Thighs	1 oz.	4	65
Shady Brook Wings	3 oz.	6	130
Whole Turkey	3.5 oz.	10	200

Soup:

Canned:

Food	Serving	Fat Grams	Cals
Healthy Choice Bean & Ham	7.5 oz.	4	220
Campbell Bean w/Bacon	8 oz.	4	140
College Inn Beef Broth	7 oz.	0	16
Campbell Beef Noodle	8 oz.	3	70
Lipton Beef Noodle	8 oz.	Trace	85
Goya Black Bean	7.5 oz.	4	160
Gold's Borscht	8 oz.	0	100
Health Valley Chicken Broth	7.5 oz.	2	35
Campbell Chicken Corn Chowder	11 oz.	21	340
Pritikin Lentil	7 oz.	0	100

Food	Serving	Fat Grams	Cals
Snow's Clam Chowder	7.5 oz.	2	70
Health Valley Minestrone	7.5 oz.	3	130
American New England Chowder	4 oz.	6	145
Pritikin Split Pea	7.5 oz.	Trace	130
Campbell Tomato 2% milk	8 oz.	2	90
Campbell Vegetable	8 oz.	2	90

Vegetables:

Mixed, Frozen:

Food	Serving	Fat Grams	Cals
Hanover broccoli, cauliflower	½ cup	0	20
Broccoli, cauliflower, carrots with cheese sauce	½ cup	6	89
Chinese stir fry	½ cup	Trace	36
Japanese stir fry	½ cup	Trace	29
Mixed vegetables w/onion	⅓ cup	5	97
Oriental blend	½ cup	0	25
Peas, onions, cheese sauce	½ cup	6	126
Stew vegetables	3 oz.	Trace	50
Peas & onions cooked	½ cup	Trace	40
Fresh zucchini	½ oz.	Trace	3
Canned tomatoes	½ cup	Trace	40
Canned spinach	½ cup	0	25
Fresh shallots, chopped	1 tbsp	Trace	7
Sauerkraut, canned	½ cup	0	20
Fresh baked potato	5 oz.	Trace	220
Canned peas	½ cup	0	90
Canned corn	½ cup	0	70
Canned carrots	½ cup	0	20

Food	Serving	Fat Grams	Cals
Yogurt:			
Cabot all flavors	8 oz.	3	220
Apples 'N Spice No-fat	8 oz.	Trace	190
Black Cherry Classic	8 oz.	6	230
Colombo Blueberry Classic	8 oz.	6	230
Dannon Blueberry No-fat	8 oz.	0	100
Yoplait Blueberry Original	6 oz.	3	190
Knudsen Lemon w/Aspartame	8 oz.	0	70
La Yogurt Peach	6 oz.	4	190
Mountain High Plain	8 oz.	9	200
Meadow Gold Raspberry Sundae	8 oz.	4	250
New Country Strawberry	6 oz.	2	150

Three Steps to Flatten Your Belly

Appendix

12 Monthly Exercise and Aerobic Charts

Date	Warm	1	2	3	4	5	6	7	8	9	10	11	12	13	14	15	16	17	18	19	20	21	22	23	24	Cool	Type	Time	Weight
											EXERCISE #			LEVEL___													AEROBICS		
1																													
2																													
3																													
4																													
5																													
6																													
7																													
8																													
9																													
10																													
11																													
12																													
13																													
14																													
15																													
16																													
17																													
18																													
19																													
20																													
21																													
22																													
23																													
24																													
25																													
26																													
27																													
28																													
29																													
30																													
31																													

Development Levels: #1-4 reps, #2-6 reps, #3- 8 resp, #4-10 reps, #5-12 reps, #6-16 reps, #7-18 reps, #8-20 reps, #9-22 reps, #10-24 reps

| | | EXERCISE # LEVEL___ | | | | | | | | | | | | | | | | | | | | | | | | | AEROBICS | | |
Date	Warm	1	2	3	4	5	6	7	8	9	10	11	12	13	14	15	16	17	18	19	20	21	22	23	24	Cool	Type	Time	Weight
1																													
2																													
3																													
4																													
5																													
6																													
7																													
8																													
9																													
10																													
11																													
12																													
13																													
14																													
15																													
16																													
17																													
18																													
19																													
20																													
21																													
22																													
23																													
24																													
25																													
26																													
27																													
28																													
29																													
30																													
31																													

Development Levels: #1-4 reps, #2-6 reps, #3- 8 resp, #4-10 reps, #5-12 reps, #6-16 reps, #7-18 reps, #8-20 reps, #9-22 reps, #10-24 reps

Date	Warm	1	2	3	4	5	6	7	8	9	10	11	12	13	14	15	16	17	18	19	20	21	22	23	24	Cool	Type	Time	Weight
1																														
2																														
3																														
4																														
5																														
6																														
7																														
8																														
9																														
10																														
11																														
12																														
13																														
14																														
15																														
16																														
17																														
18																														
19																														
20																														
21																														
22																														
23																														
24																														
25																														
26																														
27																														
28																														
29																														
30																														
31																														

EXERCISE #   LEVEL ___   AEROBICS

151

Development Levels: #1-4 reps, #2-6 reps, #3- 8 resp, #4-10 reps, #5-12 reps, #6-16 reps, #7-18 reps, #8-20 reps, #9-22 reps, #10-24 reps

		EXERCISE #	LEVEL																								AEROBICS		
Date	Warm	1	2	3	4	5	6	7	8	9	10	11	12	13	14	15	16	17	18	19	20	21	22	23	24	Cool	Type	Time	Weight
1																													
2																													
3																													
4																													
5																													
6																													
7																													
8																													
9																													
10																													
11																													
12																													
13																													
14																													
15																													
16																													
17																													
18																													
19																													
20																													
21																													
22																													
23																													
24																													
25																													
26																													
27																													
28																													
29																													
30																													
31																													

Development Levels: #1-4 reps, #2-6 reps, #3-8 resp, #4-10 reps, #5-12 reps, #6-16 reps, #7-18 reps, #8-20 reps, #9-22 reps, #10-24 reps

		EXERCISE #																								LEVEL___		AEROBICS		
Date	Warm	1	2	3	4	5	6	7	8	9	10	11	12	13	14	15	16	17	18	19	20	21	22	23	24	Cool	Type	Time	Weight
1																													
2																													
3																													
4																													
5																													
6																													
7																													
8																													
9																													
10																													
11																													
12																													
13																													
14																													
15																													
16																													
17																													
18																													
19																													
20																													
21																													
22																													
23																													
24																													
25																													
26																													
27																													
28																													
29																													
30																													
31																													

Development Levels: #1-4 reps, #2-6 reps, #3- 8 resp, #4-10 reps, #5-12 reps, #6-16 reps, #7-18 reps, #8-20 reps, #9-22 reps, #10-24 reps

Date	Warm	1	2	3	4	5	6	7	8	9	10	11	12	13	14	15	16	17	18	19	20	21	22	23	24	Cool	Type	Time	Weight
								EXERCISE #						LEVEL													AEROBICS		
1																														
2																														
3																														
4																														
5																														
6																														
7																														
8																														
9																														
10																														
11																														
12																														
13																														
14																														
15																														
16																														
17																														
18																														
19																														
20																														
21																														
22																														
23																														
24																														
25																														
26																														
27																														
28																														
29																														
30																														
31																														

Development Levels: #1-4 reps, #2-6 reps, #3- 8 resp, #4-10 reps, #5-12 reps, #6-16 reps, #7-18 reps, #8-20 reps, #9-22 reps, #10-24 reps

AEROBICS

Date	Warm	1	2	3	4	5	6	7	8	9	10	11	12	13	14	15	16	17	18	19	20	21	22	23	24	Cool	Type	Time	Weight
										EXERCISE #		LEVEL___																	
1																													
2																													
3																													
4																													
5																													
6																													
7																													
8																													
9																													
10																													
11																													
12																													
13																													
14																													
15																													
16																													
17																													
18																													
19																													
20																													
21																													
22																													
23																													
24																													
25																													
26																													
27																													
28																													
29																													
30																													
31																													

155

Development Levels: #1-4 reps, #2-6 reps, #3- 8 resp, #4-10 reps, #5-12 reps, #6-16 reps, #7-18 reps, #8-20 reps, #9-22 reps, #10-24 reps

		EXERCISE # LEVEL																									AEROBICS		
Date	Warm	1	2	3	4	5	6	7	8	9	10	11	12	13	14	15	16	17	18	19	20	21	22	23	24	Cool	Type	Time	Weight
1																													
2																													
3																													
4																													
5																													
6																													
7																													
8																													
9																													
10																													
11																													
12																													
13																													
14																													
15																													
16																													
17																													
18																													
19																													
20																													
21																													
22																													
23																													
24																													
25																													
26																													
27																													
28																													
29																													
30																													
31																													

Development Levels: #1-4 reps, #2-6 reps, #3- 8 resp, #4-10 reps, #5-12 reps, #6-16 reps, #7-18 reps, #8-20 reps, #9-22 reps, #10-24 reps

EXERCISE #   LEVEL____

AEROBICS

Date	Warm	1	2	3	4	5	6	7	8	9	10	11	12	13	14	15	16	17	18	19	20	21	22	23	24	Cool	Type	Time	Weight
1																													
2																													
3																													
4																													
5																													
6																													
7																													
8																													
9																													
10																													
11																													
12																													
13																													
14																													
15																													
16																													
17																													
18																													
19																													
20																													
21																													
22																													
23																													
24																													
25																													
26																													
27																													
28																													
29																													
30																													
31																													

Development Levels: #1-4 reps, #2-6 reps, #3- 8 resp, #4-10 reps, #5-12 reps, #6-16 reps, #7-18 reps, #8-20 reps, #9-22 reps, #10-24 reps

157

Date	Warm	1	2	3	4	5	6	7	8	9	10	11	12	13	14	15	16	17	18	19	20	21	22	23	24	Cool	Type	Time	Weight

EXERCISE #   LEVEL___   AEROBICS

Rows for dates 1 through 31.

Development Levels: #1-4 reps, #2-6 reps, #3- 8 resp, #4-10 reps, #5-12 reps, #6-16 reps, #7-18 reps, #8-20 reps, #9-22 reps, #10-24 reps

158

AEROBICS

EXERCISE # LEVEL___

Date	Warm	1	2	3	4	5	6	7	8	9	10	11	12	13	14	15	16	17	18	19	20	21	22	23	24	Cool	Type	Time	Weight
1																														
2																														
3																														
4																														
5																														
6																														
7																														
8																														
9																														
10																														
11																														
12																														
13																														
14																														
15																														
16																														
17																														
18																														
19																														
20																														
21																														
22																														
23																														
24																														
25																														
26																														
27																														
28																														
29																														
30																														
31																														

159

Development Levels: #1-4 reps, #2-6 reps, #3- 8 resp, #4-10 reps, #5-12 reps, #6-16 reps, #7-18 reps, #8-20 reps, #9-22 reps, #10-24 reps

Date	Warm	1	2	3	4	5	6	7	8	9	10	11	12	13	14	15	16	17	18	19	20	21	22	23	24	Cool	Type	Time	Weight
													EXERCISE # LEVEL ___															**AEROBICS**	
1																													
2																													
3																													
4																													
5																													
6																													
7																													
8																													
9																													
10																													
11																													
12																													
13																													
14																													
15																													
16																													
17																													
18																													
19																													
20																													
21																													
22																													
23																													
24																													
25																													
26																													
27																													
28																													
29																													
30																													
31																													

Development Levels: #1-4 reps, #2-6 reps, #3- 8 resp, #4-10 reps, #5-12 reps, #6-16 reps, #7-18 reps, #8-20 reps, #9-22 reps, #10-24 reps

160

NOTES

NOTES

NOTES

NOTES

Other Book of Interest from United Research Publishers

The Complete Handbook of Health Tips	$12.95
How to Meet People and Make Friends	$12.95
Your Prostate: What Every Man Over 40 Needs to Know, Now!	$12.95
The Complete Handbook of U.S. Government Benefits	$12.95
Living Easy in Mexico	$12.95
Write Perfect Letters for Any Occasion	$12.95

To order, send $12.95 for each book (post paid) to:

United Research Publishers
P.O. Box 2344
Leucadia, CA 92024

To Order Additional Copies
of this Book,
Write to:

United Research Publishers
Box 2344
Leucadia, CA 92024